T0260562

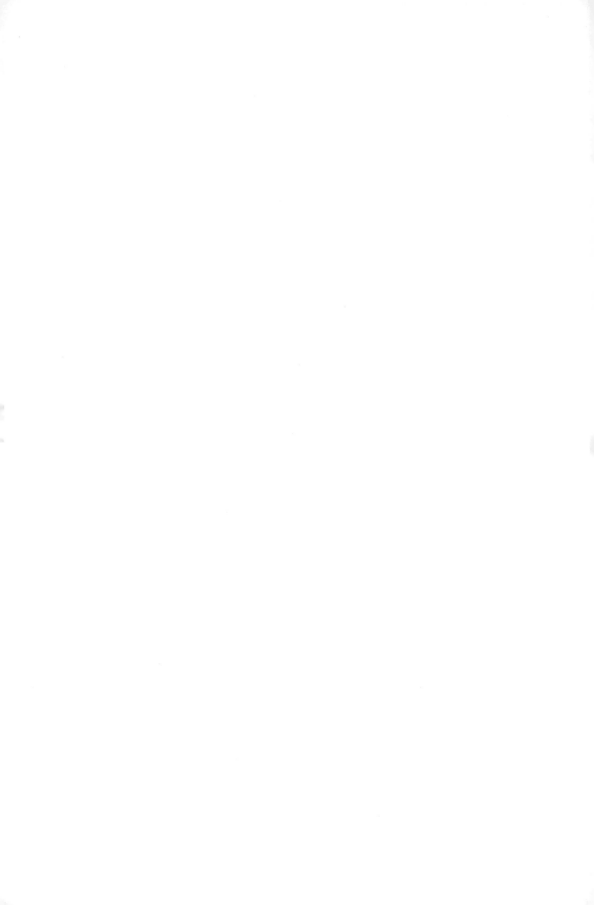

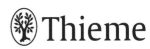

Video Atlas of Neurophysiological Monitoring in Surgery of Infiltrating Brain Tumors

Michael Sabel, MD, PhD
Professor, Head of the Center for Neurooncology
Department of Neurosurgery
University Hospital Düsseldorf
Düsseldorf, Germany

With contributions by:

Marcel Alexander Kamp
Marion Rapp
Silvio Sarubbo
Maria Smuga

106 Illustrations

Thieme
Stuttgart • New York • Delhi • Rio de Janeiro

Library of Congress Cataloging-in-Publication Data is available from the publisher.

Illustrations: Mara Gluszak and Renate Diener

Important note: Medicine is an ever-changing science undergoing continual development. Research and clinical experience are continually expanding our knowledge, in particular our knowledge of proper treatment and drug therapy. Insofar as this book mentions any dosage or application, readers may rest assured that the authors, editors, and publishers have made every effort to ensure that such references are in accordance with **the state of knowledge at the time of production of the book.**

Nevertheless, this does not involve, imply, or express any guarantee or responsibility on the part of the publishers in respect to any dosage instructions and forms of applications stated in the book. **Every user is requested to examine carefully** the manufacturers' leaflets accompanying each drug and to check, if necessary in consultation with a physician or specialist, whether the dosage schedules mentioned therein or the contraindications stated by the manufacturers differ from the statements made in the present book. Such examination is particularly important with drugs that are either rarely used or have been newly released on the market. Every dosage schedule or every form of application used is entirely at the user's own risk and responsibility. The authors and publishers request every user to report to the publishers any discrepancies or inaccuracies noticed. If errors in this work are found after publication, errata will be posted at www.thieme.com on the product description page.

Some of the product names, patents, and registered designs referred to in this book are in fact registered trademarks or proprietary names even though specific reference to this fact is not always made in the text. Therefore, the appearance of a name without designation as proprietary is not to be construed as a representation by the publisher that it is in the public domain.

Thieme addresses people of all gender identities equally. We encourage our authors to use gender-neutral or gender-equal expressions wherever the context allows.

© 2022. Thieme. All rights reserved.

Georg Thieme Verlag KG
Rüdigerstrasse 14, 70469 Stuttgart, Germany
+49 [0]711 8931 421, customerservice@thieme.de

Cover design: © Thieme
Cover image source: © Thieme
Typesetting by TNQ Technologies, India

Printed in Germany by Beltz Grafische Betriebe   5 4 3 2 1

ISBN 978-3-13-242146-2

Also available as an e-book:
eISBN 978-3-13-242147-9

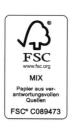

FSC
www.fsc.org
MIX
Papier aus ver-
antwortungsvollen
Quellen
FSC® C089473

To our patients.
To Professor Dr H. J. Steiger, Emeritus Professor of Neurosurgery,
University Hospital Düsseldorf, Germany

Brain surgery is a terrible profession. If I did not feel it will become different in my lifetime,
I should hate it.

– Wilder Penfield

In adult centers, the nerve paths are something fixed, ended, immutable. Everything may die,
nothing may be regenerated.

– Santiago Ramon y Cajal

Brain plasticity: a new concept in neuroscience, a new tool in neurosurgery.

–Hugues Duffau

Contents

Contents

Videos

Preface

The surgical treatment of infiltrating brain tumors is possibly the most challenging and often also the most rewarding procedure in neurosurgery. It is in the decision-making process where deep human interconnections with the patient and the relatives are build up. It is in the planning process where cutting edge neuroscience is combined with the evaluation of technical limitations, and finally, it is in the execution of the surgery where technical skills are combined with a complicated decision-making process. Despite the fact that large parts of this book deal with technical and scientific methods, this book is not about electrophysiology of the brain. It is about how to improve surgical therapy in the brain of a patient. The intention of this book is to facilitate the core process of neuro-oncology surgery, the decision to remove it or leave it, by providing the reader with the principles of a technology that enables us to make brain tumor surgery safer and more effective. Intraoperative neurophysiological monitoring is essential, but unfortunately rather complicated and not freely available technology. This book provides the basic understanding of the principles but more important is also the understanding of the practical application.

Michael Sabel, MD, PhD

Acknowledgment

We thank the staff of the University Hospital Düsseldorf for their support.

Michael Sabel, MD, PhD

Contributors

Marcel Alexander Kamp, MD, PhD
Consultant Neurosurgeon
Department of Neurosurgery
University Hospital Jena
Jena, Germany

Marion Rapp, MD, PhD
Deputy Head of the Center for Neurooncology
Department of Neurosurgery
University Hospital Düsseldorf
Düsseldorf, Germany

Michael Sabel, MD, PhD
Professor, Head of the Center for Neurooncology
Department of Neurosurgery
University Hospital Düsseldorf
Düsseldorf, Germany

Silvio Sarubbo, MD, PhD
Head of the Department of Neurosurgery
Azienda Provinciale per i Servizi Sanitari
"S. Chiara" Hospital
Trento, Italy

Maria Smuga, MTA-F
Department of Neurosurgery
University Hospital Düsseldorf
Düsseldorf, Germany

Part A

Introduction

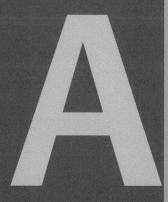

1 The Scope of This Book

First of all, this book is written by a neurosurgeon for the neurosurgical education in the field of neurooncological neurosurgery and therefore follows a strict neurosurgical perspective, focused on the practical application. So, should you expect another highly theoretical book, you will be disappointed.

Due to the increased importance of aggressive resection for the treatment of infiltrating brain tumors, the demand for neurophysiological intraoperative monitoring has dramatically increased. Unfortunately, most, if not all, neurosurgical departments lack a formal educational concept in this field. Available textbooks are very scientific and very theoretically oriented and drown you in sophisticated but in a practical sense useless information. There is therefore a need for a practical guideline to the essentials of intraoperative neurophysiological monitoring (IONM).

If you want to become a good neurooncological neurosurgeon, you will need **to understand** and **apply** neurophysiological monitoring.

To understand you should learn in this book the basics of:
- Functional anatomy of the neural pathways monitored in surgery.
- The relevant neurophysiological techniques used in monitoring and mapping during brain tumor surgery.

This is important. It is however more important (and that is what this book is focusing upon) to enable you *to practically apply* neurophysiological monitoring in brain tumor surgery. We will in this book **focus** on the "IONM-USER" aspect, similar to the way most of us use a computer. Though we are all pretty efficient and capable when working with a computer, most of us lack the deeper understanding of programming. Hence, we will not teach you the basic science of neurophysiology, but show you how to practice IONM for surgical decision-making. We divided this book into a theoretical part and a practical part. For the **theoretical part** we assume that you are in your residency and though having had some training in neurophysiology in medical school you are not too much an expert in electrophysiology. As you are in a very demanding job, you will not be able to read very long textbooks. Therefore, we will try to simplify things and point out only the relevant facts. If you want to go into more depth of the subject: fine! We will provide you with the relevant links to the heavy reading.

In the **practical part** we will show you in detail how IONM for infiltrating brain tumors works. As we will work with videos you will in fact **see** the details. We will focus on teaching how to use IONM to locate and identify eloquent structures during surgery and therefore enable you to stop the resection at the right point. Despite the fact that large parts of this book deal with technical and scientific methods, this book is **not** about electrophysiology of the brain. It is about how to improve surgical therapy in the brain of a patient. We have therefore dedicated some words on the process which integrates the technical aspect with the medical and deeply human part of the kind of surgical approach. This is the basis for entering one of the most challenging surgical decision making processes in **neurooncological neurosurgery**: *remove it or leave it.*

2 The Challenge to Treat Infiltrating Brain Tumors

Why does this book focus on the monitoring of infiltrating brain tumors?

As a neurooncological neurosurgeon you will work at the interface between highly malignant tissue that must be removed and highly functional cerebral tissue that must be preserved. The fundamental problem in Neurooncological Neurosurgery is the infiltrating part of the tumor, involving an area in which highly malignant cells are (surgically) inseparable from potentially functional tissue (▶ Fig. 2.1). On the other hand, every bit of malignant tissue that you leave behind will eventually harm the patient, will shorten his life expectancy, and will in due course cause neurological deficits and diminish the quality of life.

Therefore, surgical treatment of an infiltrating brain tumor is always a problematic trade-off between preservation of function and extent of resection (▶ Fig. 2.2). Even with the best monitoring, there are many areas where an uncertainty remains and you will need to make some difficult decisions.

The reason why IONM has gained so much importance is that the resection of infiltrating brain tumors has become the central treatment option for these lesions. Though until recently the role of resection was debated, we now have irrevocable evidence that resection has a substantial impact on overall survival of patients suffering from low-grade gliomas, high-grade gliomas, and cerebral metastases. In the following we will briefly review the data on resection. For clarification, we need to distinguish between **lesionectomy** and a resection beyond the margin of the magnetic resonance imaging (MRI)-defined lesion: the **supramarginal approach.**

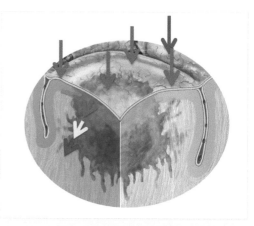

Fig. 2.2 Cortical and subcortical mapping of functionality in relation to the extent of tumor tissue. *Red*: highly functional areas; no resection possible. *Green*: not functional, resectable. *Yellow*: some uncertainty, ambiguous findings by stimulation. Might be (un)resectable.

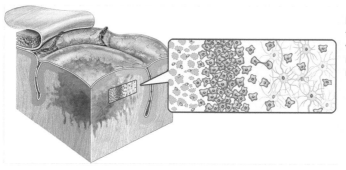

Fig. 2.1 The principal problem in treating infiltrating brain tumors: within the infiltration zone highly malignant cells are surgically inseparable from functional tissue.

3 The Impact of Lesionectomy on the Prognosis of Infiltrating Intracerebral Tumors

3.1 Evidence for Surgical Resection of Malignant Intracerebral Tumors

The role of cytoreductive surgery and complete or even supramarginal surgical resection of infiltrating cerebral tumors is of utmost importance. Therefore, we will briefly review the existing evidence for surgical resection of low- and high-grade gliomas as well as cerebral metastases.

3.2 Low-Grade Gliomas

As low-grade gliomas have the very real potential of malignant transformation to high-grade gliomas, they need to be considered as functional glioblastoma multiformes (GBMs) (▶ Fig. 3.1) and need to be considered as a precancerous condition as they exhibit a highly infiltrative growth pattern with a diffuse infiltration of still functional brain areas.[1] Therefore, a biological complete resection is likely not possible. If biological complete resection is not possible, does a radical tumor resection of low-grade gliomas translate into an improved prognosis at all? Prospective, randomized, and controlled trials addressing this question are not yet available. However, several retrospective studies suggest a benefit of a radical surgical resection of low-grade gliomas.[2,3,4,5,6,7,8,9,10,11] In a population-based parallel

cohort analysis of low-grade gliomas in patients from two different Scandinavian hospitals, overall survival after early surgical resection was significantly improved as compared to a biopsy and a "wait-and-watch" strategy.[11,12] In a retrospective analysis of over 1000 French low-grade gliomas patients, surgical resection translated into increased malignant progression-free and overall survival following extensive surgical resection.[13,14] A recent Dutch study with 228 adult patients with WHO II supratentorial gliomas identified the residual tumor volume after resection as a strong predictor for the overall survival.[15] These results confirm earlier evidence where the postoperative tumor volume was a prognostic factor of both the progression-free and overall survival.[16,17] Current guidelines advocate, therefore, extensive surgical resection as first therapeutic option.[18,19] However, postoperative neurologic deficits are a negative prognostic factor. Therefore, surgery should prevent new perisurgical deficits and a sustained quality of life of patients has a priority over maximization of surgical resection.[19]

3.3 High-Grade Gliomas

Compared to low-grade gliomas, malignant gliomas are similarly highly infiltrating but show a worse prognosis. Evidence for cytoreductive surgery for malignant gliomas was demonstrated in

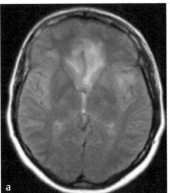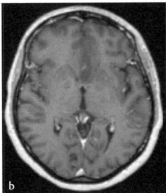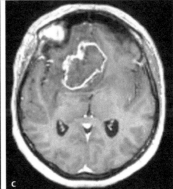

Fig. 3.1 (a-c) Malignant transformation of a (after magnetic resonance imaging [MRI] criteria) low-grade glioma into a high-grade glioma 15 months after diagnosis of the lesion.

retrospective and prospective studies:[20] The beneficial effect of a surgical resection as compared to a biopsy alone was demonstrated already in the 1950s and in two later prospective studies.[21,22,23] Moreover, the post-hoc analysis of the prospective randomized and controlled 5-amino-laevulinic acid (5-ALA) study with 270 glioblastoma patients comparing conventional with 5-ALA fluorescence-guided resection identified the postoperative tumor volume as prognostic factor for the overall survival.[24,25] The later prospective, randomized, and controlled single-center iMRI study with 58 glioblastoma patients analyzed the impact of the use of an intraoperative MRI guidance on extent of resection. As in the 5-ALA study, the more complete tumor resections in the study group translated in a significantly prolonged progression-free survival.[24,26] However, the iMRI was neither designed nor powered for a further analysis of a potential effect of extent of surgical resection on overall survival.[27] Based on these data, complete surgical resection of malignant gliomas (if feasible) is standard of care and recommended by the current guidelines.[26] Again, although complete surgical resection of malignant gliomas should be aimed at, the preservation of the patient's neurologic integrity is prior to the maximization of surgical resection.[19]

3.4 Cerebral Metastases

In contrast to low- and high-grade gliomas, cerebral metastases are more sharply delimitated from the adjacent brain tissue. Nevertheless, most metastases have the properties of albeit limited, but still relevant, local brain infiltration.[27,28,29,30] Therefore, treatment of cerebral metastases should aim at the resection of this limited infiltration zone and therefore aim at a local cure. Evidence for a surgical resection of one to four cerebral metastases have been established from phase III studies from the 1990s comparing whole-brain radiation therapy (WBRT) alone with surgery combined with WBRT. In particular in the studies by Patchell and by Noordijk and Vecht, a combined surgical and adjuvant treatment was associated with a significantly improved overall survival.[31,32,33] In nearly all more recent phase III studies, overall survival was more related to the systemic status of cancer patients than to the cranial situation.[34,35,36,37,38] However, the beneficial role of lesionectomy for a single, accessible metastasis is unquestionable. In

other words, an adequate treatment of a single cerebral metastasis by surgical resection (or single-fraction radiosurgery/irradiation) is the prerequisite to shift the prognosis of cancer patients from the cranial situation to the systemic status. However, prospective and controlled studies relating the residual tumor after surgery to the rate of local recurrences and finally to the overall survival are lacking. Nevertheless, retrospective studies suggest such an association.[39] Furthermore, extension of surgical resection toward a supramarginal resection might additionally result in a better local control as compared to conventional metastectomy.[28,40,41,42,43,44,45] In conclusion, at least complete surgical resection of a single cerebral metastasis is together with single-fraction radiosurgery the first therapeutic option and advocated by the actual guidelines.[46,47,48]

References

[1] Osswald M, Jung E, Sahm F, et al. Brain tumour cells interconnect to a functional and resistant network. Nature. 2015; 528(7580):93–98

[2] Duffau H, Lopes M, Arthuis F, et al. Contribution of intraoperative electrical stimulations in surgery of low grade gliomas: a comparative study between two series without (1985–96) and with (1996–2003) functional mapping in the same institution. J Neurol Neurosurg Psychiatry. 2005; 76(6):845–851

[3] Yeh SA, Ho JT, Lui CC, Huang YJ, Hsiung CY, Huang EY. Treatment outcomes and prognostic factors in patients with supratentorial low-grade gliomas. Br J Radiol. 2005; 78 (927):230–235

[4] McGirt MJ, Chaichana KL, Attenello FJ, et al. Extent of surgical resection is independently associated with survival in patients with hemispheric infiltrating low-grade gliomas. Neurosurgery. 2008; 63(4):700–707, author reply 707–708

[5] Schomas DA, Laack NN, Brown PD. Low-grade gliomas in older patients: long-term follow-up from Mayo Clinic. Cancer. 2009; 115(17):3969–3978

[6] Schomas DA, Laack NN, Rao RD, et al. Intracranial low-grade gliomas in adults: 30-year experience with long-term follow-up at Mayo Clinic. Neuro-oncol. 2009; 11(4):437–445

[7] Youland RS, Schomas DA, Brown PD, et al. Changes in presentation, treatment, and outcomes of adult low-grade gliomas over the past fifty years. Neuro-oncol. 2013; 15 (8):1102–1110

[8] Youland RS, Khwaja SS, Schomas DA, Keating GF, Wetjen NM, Laack NN. Prognostic factors and survival patterns in pediatric low-grade gliomas over 4 decades. J Pediatr Hematol Oncol. 2013; 35(3):197–205

[9] Ius T, Isola M, Budai R, et al. Low-grade glioma surgery in eloquent areas: volumetric analysis of extent of resection and its impact on overall survival. A single-institution experience in 190 patients: clinical article. J Neurosurg. 2012; 117(6):1039–1052

[10] Gousias K, Schramm J, Simon M. Extent of resection and survival in supratentorial infiltrative low-grade gliomas: analysis of and adjustment for treatment bias. Acta Neurochir (Wien). 2014; 156(2):327–337

[11] Jakola AS, Myrmel KS, Kloster R, et al. Comparison of a strategy favoring early surgical resection vs a strategy favoring watchful waiting in low-grade gliomas. JAMA. 2012; 308 (18):1881–1888

[12] Jakola AS, Unsgård G, Myrmel KS, et al. Low grade gliomas in eloquent locations - implications for surgical strategy, survival and long term quality of life. PLoS One. 2012; 7(12): e51450

[13] Capelle L, Fontaine D, Mandonnet E, et al. French Réseau d'Étude des Gliomes. Spontaneous and therapeutic prognostic factors in adult hemispheric World Health Organization Grade II gliomas: a series of 1097 cases: clinical article. J Neurosurg. 2013; 118(6):1157–1168

[14] Pallud J, Audureau E, Blonski M, et al. Epileptic seizures in diffuse low-grade gliomas in adults. Brain. 2014; 137(Pt 2): 449–462

[15] Wijnenga MMJ, French PJ, Dubbink HJ, et al. The impact of surgery in molecularly defined low-grade glioma: an integrated clinical, radiological, and molecular analysis. Neuro-oncol. 2018; 20(1):103–112

[16] Berger MS, Deliganis AV, Dobbins J, Keles GE. The effect of extent of resection on recurrence in patients with low grade cerebral hemisphere gliomas. Cancer. 1994; 74(6): 1784–1791

[17] Smith JS, Chang EF, Lamborn KR, et al. Role of extent of resection in the long-term outcome of low-grade hemispheric gliomas. J Clin Oncol. 2008; 26(8):1338–1345

[18] Soffietti R, Baumert BG, Bello L, et al. European Federation of Neurological Societies. Guidelines on management of low-grade gliomas: report of an EFNS-EANO Task Force. Eur J Neurol. 2010; 17(9):1124–1133

[19] Weller M, van den Bent M, Tonn JC, et al. European Association for Neuro-Oncology (EANO) Task Force on Gliomas. European Association for Neuro-Oncology (EANO) guideline on the diagnosis and treatment of adult astrocytic and oligodendroglial gliomas. Lancet Oncol. 2017; 18(6):e315–e329

[20] Stummer W, Kamp MA. The importance of surgical resection in malignant glioma. Curr Opin Neurol. 2009; 22(6): 645–649

[21] Laws ER, Parney IF, Huang W, et al. Glioma Outcomes Investigators. Survival following surgery and prognostic factors for recently diagnosed malignant glioma: data from the Glioma Outcomes Project. J Neurosurg. 2003; 99(3): 467–473

[22] Vuorinen V, Hinkka S, Färkkilä M, Jääskeläinen J. Debulking or biopsy of malignant glioma in elderly people: a randomised study. Acta Neurochir (Wien). 2003; 145(1):5–10

[23] Toennis W, Walter W. Glioblastoma multiforme (report on 2611 cases). Acta Neurochir Suppl (Vienna). 1959; 6: 40–62

[24] Stummer W, Pichlmeier U, Meinel T, Wiestler OD, Zanella F, Reulen HJ, ALA-Glioma Study Group. Fluorescence-guided surgery with 5-aminolevulinic acid for resection of malignant glioma: a randomised controlled multicentre phase III trial. Lancet Oncol. 2006; 7(5):392–401

[25] Stummer W, Reulen HJ, Meinel T, et al. ALA-Glioma Study Group. Extent of resection and survival in glioblastoma multiforme: identification of and adjustment for bias. Neurosurgery. 2008; 62(3):564–576, discussion 564–576

[26] Senft C, Bink A, Franz K, Vatter H, Gasser T, Seifert V. Intraoperative MRI guidance and extent of resection in glioma surgery: a randomised, controlled trial. Lancet Oncol. 2011; 12(11):997–1003

[27] Kamp MA, Grosser P, Felsberg J, et al. 5-aminolevulinic acid (5-ALA)-induced fluorescence in intracerebral metastases: a retrospective study. Acta Neurochir (Wien). 2012; 154(2): 223–228, discussion 228

[28] Kamp MA, Slotty PJ, Cornelius JF, Steiger HJ, Rapp M, Sabel M. The impact of cerebral metastases growth pattern on neurosurgical treatment. Neurosurg Rev. 2018; 41(1):77–86

[29] Berghoff AS, Rajky O, Winkler F, et al. Invasion patterns in brain metastases of solid cancers. Neuro-oncol. 2013; 15 (12):1664–1672

[30] Siam L, Bleckmann A, Chaung HN, et al. The metastatic infiltration at the metastasis/brain parenchyma-interface is very heterogeneous and has a significant impact on survival in a prospective study. Oncotarget. 2015; 6(30):29254–29267

[31] Patchell RA, Tibbs PA, Walsh JW, et al. A randomized trial of surgery in the treatment of single metastases to the brain. N Engl J Med. 1990; 322(8):494–500

[32] Noordijk EM, Vecht CJ, Haaxma-Reiche H, et al. The choice of treatment of single brain metastasis should be based on extracranial tumor activity and age. Int J Radiat Oncol Biol Phys. 1994; 29(4):711–717

[33] Vecht CJ, Haaxma-Reiche H, Noordijk EM, et al. Treatment of single brain metastasis: radiotherapy alone or combined with neurosurgery? Ann Neurol. 1993; 33(6):583–590

[34] Brown PD, Ballman KV, Cerhan JH, et al. Postoperative stereotactic radiosurgery compared with whole brain radiotherapy for resected metastatic brain disease (NCCTG N107C/CEC·3): a multicentre, randomised, controlled, phase 3 trial. Lancet Oncol. 2017; 18(8):1049–1060

[35] Brown PD, Jaeckle K, Ballman KV, et al. Effect of radiosurgery alone vs radiosurgery with whole brain radiation therapy on cognitive function in patients with 1 to 3 brain metastases: a randomized clinical trial. JAMA. 2016; 316 (4):401–409

[36] Mahajan A, Ahmed S, McAleer MF, et al. Post-operative stereotactic radiosurgery versus observation for completely resected brain metastases: a single-centre, randomised, controlled, phase 3 trial. Lancet Oncol. 2017; 18(8):1040–1048

[37] Kocher M, Soffietti R, Abacioglu U, et al. Adjuvant whole-brain radiotherapy versus observation after radiosurgery or surgical resection of one to three cerebral metastases: results of the EORTC 22952–26001 study. J Clin Oncol. 2011; 29(2):134–141

[38] Roos DE, Smith JG, Stephens SW. Radiosurgery versus surgery, both with adjuvant whole brain radiotherapy, for solitary brain metastases: a randomised controlled trial. Clin Oncol (R Coll Radiol). 2011; 23(9):646–651

[39] Kamp MA, Rapp M, Bühner J, et al. Early postoperative magnet resonance tomography after resection of cerebral metastases. Acta Neurochir (Wien). 2015; 157(9):1573–1580

[40] Kamp MA, et al. Is it all a matter of size? Impact of maximization of surgical resection in cerebral tumors. Neurosurg Rev. 2018

[41] Yoo H, Kim YZ, Nam BH, et al. Reduced local recurrence of a single brain metastasis through microscopic total resection. J Neurosurg. 2009; 110(4):730–736

[42] Kamp MA, Dibué M, Niemann L, et al. Proof of principle: supramarginal resection of cerebral metastases in eloquent brain areas. Acta Neurochir (Wien). 2012; 154(11):1981–1986

[43] Kamp MA, Dibué M, Santacroce A, et al. The tumour is not enough or is it? Problems and new concepts in the surgery of cerebral metastases. Ecancermedicalscience. 2013; 7: 306

[44] Kamp MA, Rapp M, Slotty PJ, et al. Incidence of local in-brain progression after supramarginal resection of cerebral metastases. Acta Neurochir (Wien). 2015; 157(6):905–910, discussion 910–911

[45] Pessina F, Navarria P, Cozzi L, et al. Role of surgical resection in patients with single large brain metastases: feasibility, morbidity, and local control evaluation. World Neurosurg. 2016; 94:6–12

[46] Bhangoo SS, Linskey ME, Kalkanis SN, American Association of Neurologic Surgeons (AANS), Congress of Neurologic Surgeons (CNS). Evidence-based guidelines for the management of brain metastases. Neurosurg Clin N Am. 2011; 22(1):97–104, viii

[47] Kalkanis SN, Kondziolka D, Gaspar LE, et al. The role of surgical resection in the management of newly diagnosed brain metastases: a systematic review and evidence-based clinical practice guideline. J Neurooncol. 2010; 96(1):33–43

[48] Soffietti R, Abacioglu U, Baumert B, et al. Diagnosis and treatment of brain metastases from solid tumors: guidelines from the European Association of Neuro-Oncology (EANO). Neuro-oncol. 2017; 19(2):162–174

4 The Philosophy Behind Supramarginal Resection: Functionality Becomes the Limit

Though the role of lesionectomy for infiltrating brain tumors is now established, in many cases sole lesionectomy is not the best neurooncological neurosurgery. Obviously, due to the infiltrating nature of these lesions a local surgical cure is (for gliomas) not an option. However, in many cases we can do better than just performing a lesionectomy as the surrounding tissue might not be functional but be the matrix for short-term recurrence. An exemplary case is demonstrated in ▶ Fig. 4.1. Though a perfect resection in terms of lesionectomy was achieved, the patient presented with a local recurrence 8 months after surgery. As he had

no deficit at the time of presentation with the recurrent GBM, it is very likely that the area of the recurrence would have been resectable at the time of the first surgery without inducing functional deficits. Consequent IONM would have pushed the resection further, potentially increasing the progression-free survival. Neurooncological neurosurgery has now the task to push the resection to the functional limit, beyond the MRI, hence the flair and T2-defined lesion for the low-grade gliomas or the contrast-enhancing lesion for the high-grade gliomas and cerebral metastases (▶ Fig. 4.2). This, however, makes the use of IONM indispensable.

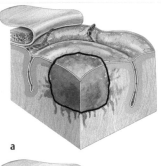
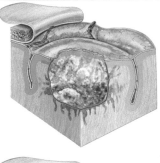

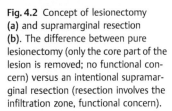
Fig. 4.1 (a, b) Typical local recurrence within 2 cm of the resection margin after 8 months. As the patient had no functional deficit at the time of recurrence, it is doubtful that the area of recurrence was functional at the time of first surgery. Supramarginal resection would probably have been possible.

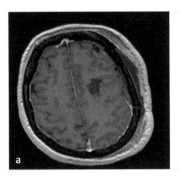
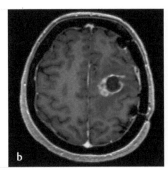
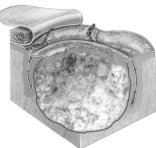
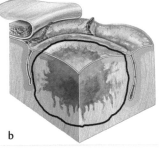

Fig. 4.2 Concept of lesionectomy (a) and supramarginal resection (b). The difference between pure lesionectomy (only the core part of the lesion is removed; no functional concern) versus an intentional supramarginal resection (resection involves the infiltration zone, functional concern).

Part B

The Theoretical Part

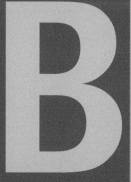

5 The Relevant Anatomy of the Functional Systems

5.1 The Scope of This Chapter

In this chapter we will review the anatomical basis of the functional systems that can routinely be tested by IONM. We will focus on the testable aspects of the motor system, the somatosensory system, the visual system, and the language system.

As the testing of higher neuropsychological functions is not yet fully established, we will not elaborate this topic in detail in this book. However, keep in mind that the patient's quality of life does not only depend on his ability to walk, talk, and see.

Do not aspect a thorough neuroanatomical review of the central nervous system (CNS); in fact, it is our intention to oversimplify things a little. It is very important that you understand that the neurosurgical application of IONM is based on a profound knowledge of the cortical as well as the subcortical localization of functions. As compared to the limited "testable" areas of the cortical surface, the complexity of the subcortical functional pathways is immense. The increased understanding of the subcortical pathways has direct impact on surgical strategies: in addition to topological (cortical) interference with functions, the neurosurgeon is also interfering with the subcortical pathways (hodos, ancient Greek word for "road travelled"). Therefore, both topological und hodological aspects of functionality must be integrated into surgical planning strategies which extend the concept of pure cortical localization of functions to the complex subcortical functional systems (▶ Fig. 5.1). For the mapping of cortical and subcortical functional structures, you need to mentally visualize these structures as you plan the approach and build up a road map of the test you need to employ. In the following chapter we will focus on this aspect of functional anatomy: the three-dimensional localization of testable functions.

5.2 Cortical Anatomy

Cortical functionality might be correlated to specific structural neuronal organization.

Brodmann areas (▶ Fig. 5.2) are cortical areas with specific neuronal cytoarchitecture. Some of these structural features correlate with cortical functions. For example, Brodmann areas 1, 2, and 3 are the primary somatosensory cortex; area 4 is the primary motor cortex; area 17 is the primary visual cortex; and areas 41 and 42 correspond closely to primary auditory cortex. Higher cognitive functions are also consistently localized to the same Brodmann areas. Broca's speech and language area correspond, (i.e., to Brodmann areas 44 and 45). It is however important to note, that, though the correlation of structural cortical features is of great

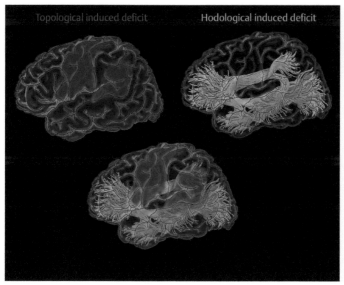

Topological induced deficit   Hodological induced deficit

Fig. 5.1 Integrated cortical and subcortical functional approach. When planning a resection both cortical and subcortical functionality must be identified and preserved.

neuroscientific interest,[1] the functionality of these areas can only be fully appreciated when correlated to the connectivity of these areas within the neuronal networks, the human connectome (▶ Fig. 5.1). Therefore, functionality of a brain region can only be defined if cortical and subcortical functionalities are analyzed, hence the importance of intraoperative of cortical and subcortical testing (Chapter B4).

5.2.1 Lobes

In ▶ Fig. 5.3 we outline a useful simplification of the cerebral lobes: frontal, temporal, parietal, occipital.

The nomenclature and anatomical position of the gyri and sulci are demonstrated in ▶ Fig. 5.4 based on the human brain template, MNI ICBM152, with modifications from Tate et al.[2]

For the identification of cortical functional areas and correlation with the subcortical system, a cortical parcellation system (CPS) as suggested by Corina et al is useful.[3] This system divides the cortical surface into 37 regions (▶ Fig. 5.5).

Superior, medial, and inferior frontal gyri are each divided into rostral, anterior, medial, and posterior segments. Similarly, the temporal lobes are divided into superior, medial, and inferior temporal lobe, again divided into rostral, anterior, medial,

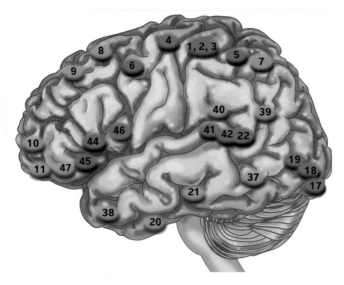

Fig. 5.2 Brodmann areas of the brain. *Areas in blue*: distinct cytoarchitectural areas, which correlate with clinical, intraoperatively testable functions.

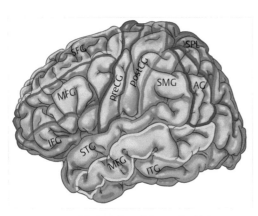

Fig. 5.3 A simplified outline of the cerebral lobes: frontal, temporal, parietal, occipital.

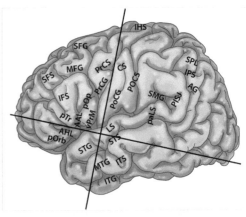

Fig. 5.4 The nomenclature and anatomical position of the gyri and sulci are demonstrated based on the human brain template, MNI ICBM152.[2]

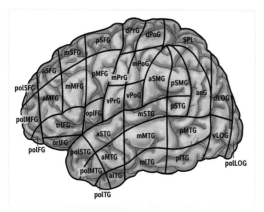

Fig. 5.5 A detailed division of the cortical surface into 37 regions suggested by Corina et al.[3]

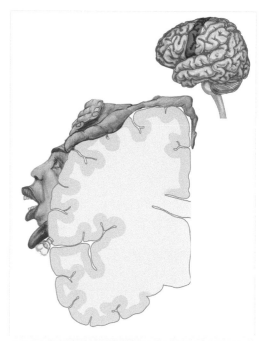

Fig. 5.6 Topological-functional orientation of the motor cortex. Note that direct cortical stimulation of motor language areas necessitates an exposure close to the Sylvian fissure. For direct cortical stimulation of the leg an interhemispheric exposure is needed.

and posterior segments. In the central region pre- and postcentral lobe are divided into superior, medial, and inferior. Posterior to these is the medial located superior parietal lobe and inferior parietal lobe composed by the anterior and posterior supramarginal gyrus (SMG) and angular gyrus (AG). Again, posteriorly are the lateral superior and inferior and medial occipital lobes.

Subcortical anatomy will be described within the context of the functional systems.

5.3 Motor System

The motor system consists of the pyramidal and extrapyramidal system. We will focus on the pyramidal motor system. The pyramidal motor system starts in the motor cortex (precentral gyrus, aka M1), where the upper motor neurons are located (Betz cells). The motor impulses are originated in these giant pyramidal cells. The axons of these cells pass through the corona radiata and then through the genu and anterior third of the internal capsule and continue to descend in the midbrain and the medulla oblongata. From a surgical point of view, the topological and functional orientation of the motor cortex and the corticospinal/bulbar tract are of utmost importance (▶ Fig. 5.6). For practical purposes it is important to note that the cortical presentation of the leg is "hidden" in the interhemispheric fissure and that the area of throat and tongue is located just superior to the Sylvian fissure. So, if you want to directly stimulate these cortical areas you need to enter the interhemispheric fissure for the leg and need to

expose the brain up to the Sylvian fissure for motor components of language (see also Section 7.5). As for the fiber tracts: The cortical spinal and corticobulbar fibers also have a topological order (▶ Fig. 5.7). The corticobulbar and the corticospinal tract descend separately through the genu and the anterior third of the posterior limb of the internal capsule. The corticospinal tracts are organized along a long axis. Hand fibers are located anteromedial to foot fibers. For subcortical stimulation you may imagine a trajectory from the cortical presentation of functions to the internal capsule: an almost perpendicular medial course for the leg and a more horizontal lateral course for the tracts from face and arm (▶ Fig. 5.7).

5.4 The Somatosensory System

The somatosensory system relays sensory information from the periphery ultimately to the sensory cortex.

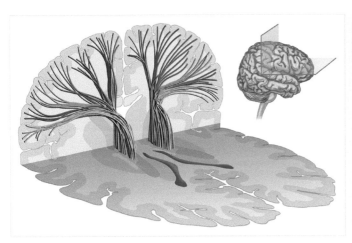

Fig. 5.7 The topological order of the cortical-spinal tract: Hand fibers are located anteromedial to foot fibers.

Sensation-induced nerve impulses travel via a three-neuron system through the spinal cord, brainstem, and thalamus to the sensory cortex in the parietal lobe. We will discuss here the anatomy relevant for the understanding of the somatosensory-evoked potentials (SSEPs.). The first thing to note is that the somatosensory system has a very long course through important, even essential neuronal structures (i.e., brain stem) and is therefore a good indicator for potential impairment of these structures. In more detail: Sensory input is carried to the dorsal root ganglia, where the first-order neurons are located (▶ Fig. 5.8). The signal is transferred into the spinal cord and runs through the posterior column-medial lemniscus pathway via gracilis (T7 and below) or cuneatus (T6 and above). The signal is then, depending on the type of stimulus, processed by second-order neurons. The spinothalamic tract and the medial lemniscus transport the signal through the basal part of the tegmentum in the pons and midbrain until they reach the thalamus. In the thalamus, they connect with the third-order neurons in the ventral posterior lateral (VPL) nucleus. The trigeminal lemniscus (face) synapses in the ventral posterior medial (VPM) nucleus. From the thalamus, the signals are projected to the cortical sensory areas, where information is integrated and analyzed.

Clinical application: As SSEPs correspond to an electrical volley at different (ascending) levels, the localization of an injury at the spinal, brainstem, and internal capsule level can be estimated (▶ Fig. 5.8).

The primary somatosensory cortex is located in the postcentral gyrus (Brodmann areas 1, 2, and 3, commonly referred to as S1, ▶ Fig. 5.9). S1 is connected with the motor cortex, somatosensory association cortex, and the contralateral S1. Similar to the primary motor cortex, the primary somatosensory cortex is topologically organized. Leg fibers are located medially, whereas arm, hand, face, and tongue fibers are on the lateral surface of the somatosensory area. Body areas particularly important to the sensory system (e.g., the face, lips, and hand) are given larger representation than other areas (▶ Fig. 5.9).

Clinical application: Stimulation with a 60-Hz bipolar stimulator in this area can induce sensory phenomena in a topological order.

5.5 Focus: Functional Aspects of Language

In this section we review the structural and functional anatomy of language.

To understand the "neurosurgical" implications of language you need to keep in mind that the functional system of language has a pure motor (executive) aspect (coordination of, i.e., throat, larynx, tongue, and lips) located in both hemispheres (▶ Fig. 5.6) and the incredibly complicated higher cognitive functions of language (located in the dominant hemisphere, usually left) in a much broader sense than just producing articulated sounds. These include conceptualization, lexical, syntax, phonological, and semantic aspects. The language system is a paradigm for anatomical functional substrates defined by (1) cortical areas and (2) subcortical connections (▶ Fig. 5.1). Though this is a book on basics and principles of IONM we will reflect on the language system

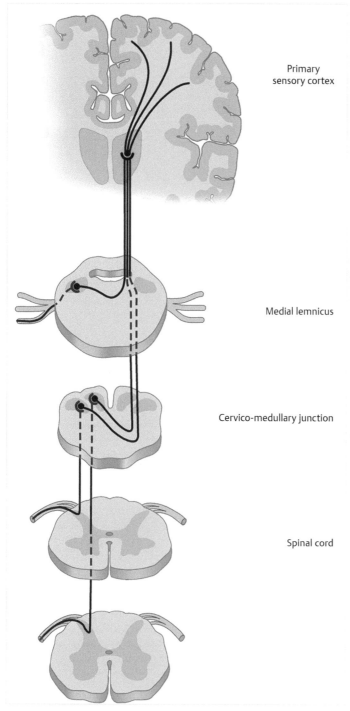

Primary
sensory cortex

Medial lemnicus

Cervico-medullary junction

Spinal cord

Fig. 5.8 The anatomy of the somato-sensory system as relevant for the understanding of the SSEPs. The disruption of the electrical volley at the different levels can indicate the localization of the injury.

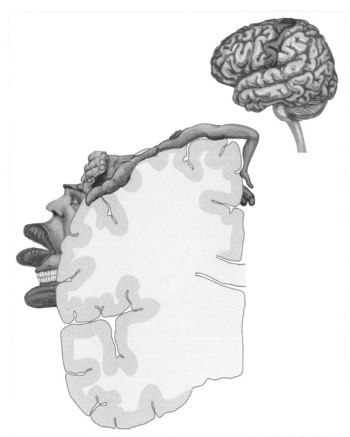

Fig. 5.9 The topological organization of the primary somatosensory cortex. Note the larger representation of face areas as compared to the extremities.

including the visual system in more detail. This is necessary because proper monitoring of the language system depends on a profound knowledge of the cortical and subcortical functional neuroanatomy and a basic understanding of the connectome.

5.5.1 Structural and Functional Anatomy

Hickok and Poeppel summarized in 2007 the evidences coming from multimodal neuroscientific studies about the organization of the language network in the human brain.[4] The fundamental scheme includes a dual-stream model (▸ Fig. 5.10 and ▸ Fig. 5.11). The dorsal stream is substantially dedicated to the codification of sensory input into articulatory movements, and the ventral stream is dedicated in decoding sensory input into semantic contents.

The integration between these two basic functional routes subserves the semantic and nonsemantic comprehension of every sensory (e.g., auditory, visual, somatosensory) input to the human brain, and produce the language planning and output, with a continuous feedforward/feedback regulation by those or other input. Finally, the structure of the phrase (meaning and conceptual links between words) is constructed by the syntactic network (including the lexicon of items and the system to combine them, or more schematically: words and grammar for combining these). The dorsal pathways connect the main hubs for syntactic elaboration, comprehensively: inferior frontal gyrus (IFG) (Pars Op and Ptri), posterior temporal lobe (i.e., posterior middle temporal gyrus [pMTG] and posterior superior temporal gyrus [pSTG]) and inferior parietal lobule (IPL, in particular, AG and SMG)[6] (▸ Fig. 5.11).

Even considering just these three submodalities (i.e., semantic, phonological, syntactic) and their

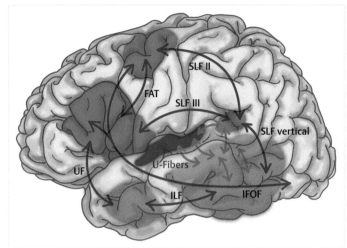

Fig. 5.10 The main connections of the dual-stream model of language processing. Modified from the original scheme by Hickok and Poeppel[5]. A schematic distribution of cortical epicenters of dorsal (in *blue*) and ventral (*green*) streams, and of the main sensory-integration areas (*orange, violet,* and *red*) with the different bundles connecting these (FAT, frontal aslant tract; IFOF, inferior fronto-occipital fascicle; ILF, inferior longitudinal fascicle; SLF, superior longitudinal fascicle; UF, uncinate fascicle).

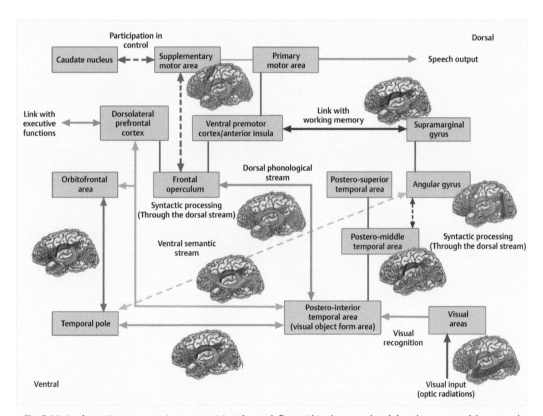

Fig. 5.11 A schematic representation summarizing the work flow within the ventral and dorsal stream model proposed by Hickok and Poeppel.[4]

own working memories, the language network was demonstrated as one of the most distributed networks at individual and interindividual levels (► Fig. 5.12a, b).[7]

Recently, more and more evidences have confirmed this fundamental organization. Especially, direct electrical stimulation (DES) brain mapping data has improved our knowledge about the structural organization of different parallel subnetworks, and the intricate maze of input/output integration and language elaboration and production.[10,11,12] In fact, different long-range bundles or subcomponents of those in the dorsal (i.e., perisylvian) and

ventral white matter of the human brain were demonstrated to play specialized roles in the different submodalities of functional processing explorable during surgery, according to the schematic reproduction reported in ► Fig. 5.13a, b.

Basically, the dorsal stream (and the bundles included in it) is specialized in phonological and syntactic elaboration and articulatory planning, and the ventral stream in semantic processing. These two systems are highly integrated at cortical and subcortical levels by means of short fibers connecting critical cortical epicenters at the temporo-parieto-occipital junction and in the

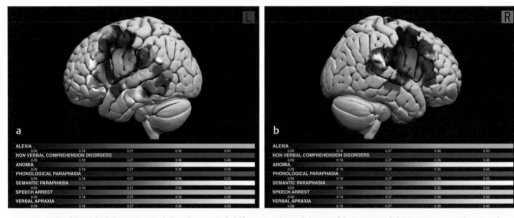

Fig. 5.12 (a, b) Probabilistic cortical distribution of different submodalities of language elaboration, according to the direct electrical stimulation atlas recently published by Sarubbo et al[8 9] in the left **(a)** and right **(b)** hemisphere.

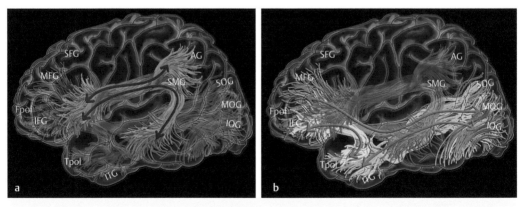

Fig. 5.13 (a) Schematic representation of the dorsal (SLF III and AF, respectively, *long and short purple arrow*) and **(b)** ventral long (IFOF, *long yellow arrow*) and midrange (ILF and UF, respectively, *long and short yellow arrow*) providing a multilobe and high-distributed connection for phonological, semantic, and syntactic nodes dedicated to language processing (IFOF, inferior fronto-occipital fascicle; ILF, inferior longitudinal fascicle; SLF, superior longitudinal fascicle; UF, uncinate fascicle).

dorsal and ventral frontal lobes which constitute the main territories of functional interconnection between the dorsal and ventral routes.

Finally, the main sensory input for language elaboration is subserved by the projection fibers of acoustic radiation (AR) for auditory stimuli and optic radiations (ORs) for visual stimuli.

5.5.2 Sensory Input and Projection Pathways

Auditory and visual stimuli are the main sensory inputs that impact language elaboration (▶ Fig. 5.14). The primary cortices, (i.e., the Heschl gyrus (HG) and calcarine cortex), are the territories of termination of the projection pathways of the projection fibers coming from the lateral and medial geniculate body, (i.e., AR and OR), respectively, for auditory and visual inputs. The stimulation of HG is not frequent, considering the anatomical subopercular location. Nevertheless, the stimulation around the posterior Sylvian point can produce acoustic responses. Even at subcortical level the fibers of AR are rarely encountered with DES, considering the strict anatomical relationship of the arcuate fascicle (AF) with the stem (i.e., the region where the fibers are mainly concentrated and collected),[13,14] regularly eliciting phonological paraphasia and that constitute a major functional limit for pushing the resection over. This strict anatomical relationship of auditory network with the long fibers of AF and superior longitudinal fascicle (SLF) III terminating in pSTG and pMTG and the short-range connectivity

provided by the U-fibers between HG and these cortical territories, which are crucial regions for phonological and speech articulatory planning of language, is the structural background of a close functional relationship between the auditory network and the dorsal stream. It provides sound representations for phonological-motor planning of language, and a feedback control for speech production together with the somatosensory ventral areas (i.e., ventral portion of the PostCG).[15]

The primary visual cortex is distributed in the lateral, medial, superior, and inferior calcarine cortices separated from the calcarine sulcus (▶ Fig. 5.15).

OR fibers are deep seated in the white matter of the temporal lobe. A recent description of this projection pathway proposed a division into superior and inferior groups of fibers terminating, respectively, in the superior and inferior calcarine cortex, and thus competent for subserving sensory input from, respectively, the inferior and superior contralateral visual quadrants of the visual field.[16] The subdivision of this large group of fibers is particularly useful from a neurosurgical perspective, considering the chance to establish neuroanatomical and functional landmarks to assess the limit between these and, as a consequence, between the superior and inferior quadrants of the visual field.

The ventricular system is the first anatomical reference, considering the deep location of the OR in the white matter of the occipital and temporal lobes and strict relationship of the OR with the walls of this structure.[17] The inferior border of the lateral wall of the trigone constitutes a first landmark between superior and inferior OR. Proceeding anteriorly, the roof of the temporal horn

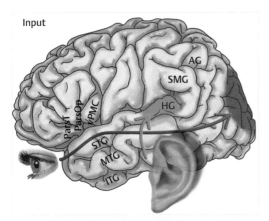

Fig. 5.14 Schematic representation of sensory (auditory and visual) input related to language elaboration. (*Long arrow*: visual input; *short arrow*: auditory input)

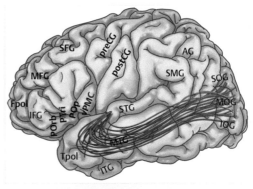

Fig. 5.15 Schematic representation of optic radiation course.

constitutes a second landmark between superior and inferior OR.[16]

Moreover, the superior OR is covered all over its course from the fibers of the inferior fronto-occipital fascicle (IFOF), a crucial structure for semantic verbal and non-verbal processing and clearly identifiable at DES subcortical mapping (▶ Fig. 5.16).[16]

5.5.3 Dorsal Stream

Basically, the dorsal stream is composed of the fibers of the dorsal longitudinal system (DLS) mainly constituted from the SLF.[18] In fact, the SLF is the prominent portion of the DLS, which connects large portions of the frontal lobe with the temporal and the parietal lobe. The most ventral

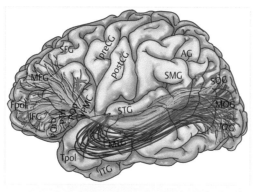

Fig. 5.16 Schematic representation of the overlapping course between the superior optic radiation and the ventral portion of inferior fronto-occipital fascicle (IFOF).

component of the SLF is usually called SLF III. This nomenclature of the different components of the SLF is derived by the nonhuman primate anatomy,[5] and it is probably reductive for the human brain but it is crucial to elucidate this for a correct identification of the different subcomponents of the different layers of human white matter,[19] especially in the perspective of a functional classification of these fibers.

However, SLF III (also known as the indirect anterior component of the SLF or horizontal portion)[20,21] is a thick layer of fibers running just below the layer of the U-fibers of the ventral frontoparietal junction and connecting the ventral premotor cortex (VPMC) and the pars opercularis (POp) of the IFG (▶ Fig. 5.17).[22] SLF III play a crucial role in connecting the cortical frontoventral and parietal epicenters specialized in the speech planning, also known as speech articulatory network speech articulatory network (SAN).

The second component of the dorsal system language processing network is the AF (▶ Fig. 5.18). AF, providing the only direct connection between the posteroventral portion of the frontal lobe (namely, the POp and triangularis [PTri] of the IFG and the posterior third of the middle frontal gyrus [MFG]) with the temporal lobe (namely, the posterior third of the STG, and the posterior and middle thirds of the MTG and the inferior temporal gyrus [ITG]), was demonstrated to be the main stream for phonological and syntactic processing. Classically the stimulation of this white matter area (deeper in respect to the SLF III at frontoparietal level) induces phonological paraphasia during object naming (e.g., visualizing a dog the patient states: "this is a frog").

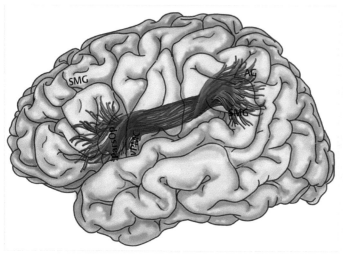

Fig. 5.17 Schematic representation of the SLF III connecting the frontal opercula (VPMC and POp) with the inferior parietal lobule (namely, AG and SMG) (AG, angular gyrus; POp, pars opercularis; SLF, superior longitudinal fascicle; SMG, supramarginal gyrus; VPMC, ventral premotor cortex).

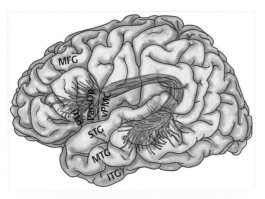

Fig. 5.18 Schematic representation of the AF fibers connecting the frontal opercula (VPMC, POp, and PTri) with STG, MTG, and ITG. (AF, arcuate fascicle; ITG: inferior temporal gyrus; MTG, middle temporal gyrus; POp, pars opercularis; PTri, pars triangularis; STG, superior temporal gyrus).

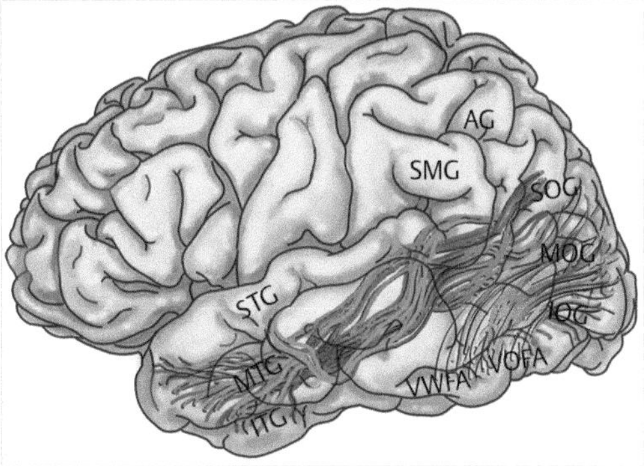

Fig. 5.19 Schematic representation of the posterior (or dorsal, in *yellow*) and anterior (or ventral, in *blue*) components of inferior longitudinal fascicle (ILF) fibers connecting the occipital cortices and the precuneus with the basal and lateral cortices of the temporal lobe and the temporal pole.

5.5.4 Ventral Stream

The ventral stream is connected by different layers of the so-called ventral longitudinal system (VLS). The main bundles with a demonstrated functional role in the verbal and nonverbal semantic processing and in the sensory integration of visual information in the language system are: the inferior longitudinal fascicle (ILF), the uncinate fascicle (UF), and the inferior fronto-occipital fascicle (IFOF).

The ILF is a long-range and multilayer bundle connecting the occipital cortices and the precuneus with the lateral and basal temporal cortices (▶ Fig. 5.19).[22,23,24] In particular, the posterior and lateral portions of the ILF connecting the posterior inferior temporal cortex (ITCp) and the anterior portion of the visual word form area (VWFA) was demonstrated to induce reading disturbances in the hemisphere specialized in language elaboration (i.e., the left, in right-handers).

Ventral to the ILF fibers, the fibers of IFOF run from the occipital cortices, cuneus, and the precuneus to the frontal lobe (▶ Fig. 5.20). The anatomical distribution of the IFOF was recently renewed considering its crucial and proved role as main stream of semantic verbal comprehension. In fact, IFOF is the longest white matter associative bundle and it can be divided in dorsal and ventral layer of fibers clearly identifiable at the level of the stem (i.e., ventral third of the external capsule) connecting, respectively, the IFG (i.e., PTri, POrb), the

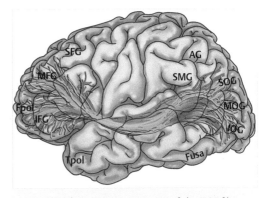

Fig. 5.20 Schematic representation of the IFOF fibers connecting the occipital and parietal cortices with the IFG, frontal pole, lateral OFC, and the middle third of the MFG and SFG (IFG, inferior frontal gyrus; IFOF, inferior fronto-occipital fascicle; MFG, middle frontal gyrus; SFG, superior frontal gyrus).

frontal pole (Fp), and lateral orbitofrontal cortex (LOFC), and the middle third of MFG and SFG (i.e., dorsolateral prefrontal cortex, DLPFC) with the parietal and occipital cortices.[22,25,26,27] Even in the hemisphere not specialized in language processing, IFOF was demonstrated crucial in connecting a distributed network processing nonverbal comprehension (e.g., semantic association troubles).[28] Typical functional responses in contact with the IFOF fibers in the hemisphere specialized in language are semantic paraphasia (visualizing a dog the patient states: "this is a cloud") or anomia (visualizing an object the patient is not able to denominate, and classically states: "this is a…") during object naming.

The last component of the ventral route is the uncinate fascicle (UF). UF is basically represented as an hook-shaped bundle of fibers connecting the temporal pole (Tp) to the frontal pole (Fp, ▶ Fig. 5.21). The structure of this layer of fibers, running between the temporal and the frontal lobe compacting in a stem just ventral to the IFOF stem (in the most ventral third of the EC), is now demonstrated to have a larger and multilayer distribution including the whole anterior third of the temporal lobe (including the mesial cortices) and the dorsal and mesial cortices of the frontal lobe.[29] Even if UF was considered for a long time a relay of the mainstream for semantic elaboration (completed at temporo-occipital level by ILF), large resection of this bundle (or at least of the main component) following temporal lobectomy induces disturbances in submodality of semantic elaboration such as recognition of famous faces.[30]

5.5.5 Dorsoventral Integration

U-fibers and midrange bundles constitute a cornerstone of the intercortical connectivity for integration of sensory input and planned output between the dorsal and the ventral stream.

The temporo-parieto-occipital junction, in fact, is the first of two crucial crisscross areas for long- and short-range connectivity subserving the complex integration of sensory stimuli (in particular, visual) in the phonological and semantic stream.[22,24] Supramarginal gyrus (SMG) and angular gyrus (AG) are also known as Geschwind Territories and constitute a crucial hub of the SAN. These cortices are strongly interconnected with the auditory cortex (namely, the HG) and the posterior two-thirds of the STG and MTG throughout a continuous and homogenous layer of U-fibers (▶ Fig. 5.22).

A deeper layer of transverse fibers including the indirect posterior portion of the SLF (also called vertical SLF) and the vertical occipital fascicle (VOF) subserve a second and midrange connectivity between cortices of the dorsal route (namely, Geschwind Territories) and more distant cortical areas including also the occipital lateral cortices (i.e., SOG, MOG, and IOG), the ITG (▶ Fig. 5.23).

Finally, deeper and longitudinal fibers of the ILF participate in this complex structural integration of language elaboration at the level of the temporo-parieto-occipital carrefour, connecting the occipital cortices to the visual object form area (VOFA, basal cortex of the posterior temporal lobe) crucial for processing visual object recognition input (▶ Fig. 5.23).

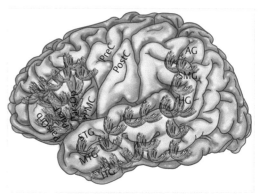

Fig. 5.22 Schematic representation of the complex architecture of the U-fibers in the temporo-parieto-occipital junction and in the ventral frontal lobe providing the shortest connections of the cortical nodes for functional processing and integration of the different submodalities of language elaboration (AG, angular gyrus; HG, Heschl gyrus; ITG, inferior temporal gyrus; MTG, middle temporal gyrus; ParOrb, pars orbitalis; ParsT, pars triangularis; ParsOp, pars opercularis; PreC, pre-central gyrus; PostC, post-central gyrus; STG, superior temporal gyrus).

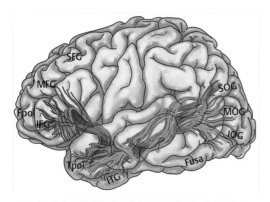

Fig. 5.21 Schematic representation of the UF fibers (in *purple*) connecting the temporal and frontal poles and completing together with the ILF (in *blue*) an indirect functional connection of the ventral stream between the temporo-occipital and frontal lobes (ILF, inferior longitudinal fascicle; UF, uncinate fascicle).

The stimulation at cortical and subcortical levels in these regions can frequently induce anomia in addition to phonological disturbances, probably due also to the dorsoventral integration deactivation induced by stimulation.[8] The structure of long- and short-range white matter in these regions and the close relationship between these fibers is crucial for planning safe functional resection as we will discuss in the chapter regarding topographical anatomy.

A second crucial area for cortical functional integration between dorsal and ventral routes is the short connectivity of the frontal lobe where the nodes of phonological, semantic, and syntactic elaboration are supported by the horizontal U-fibers connecting the frontal opercula (namely, POp, PTri, and POrb) with ventral premotor and motor cortices (namely, the ventral premotor cortex, VPMC) and the vertical U-fibers connecting these ventral areas with the dorsolateral prefrontal cortices (▶ Fig. 5.23). This complex system of U-fibers connecting the large territories of termination of all the long and midrange pathways explored (with the only exception of ILF) supports this strong integration and the continuous regulation

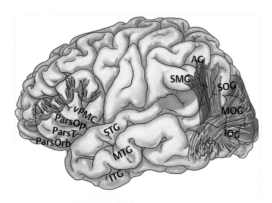

Fig. 5.23 Schematic representation of the posterior transverse layer fibers belonging to vertical SLF (or indirect posterior component of SLF, *purple*) and VOF (*green*) and the crossing longitudinal fibers of the posterior (or dorsal) component of the ILF (AG, angular gyrus; ILF, inferior longitudinal fascicle; IOG, inferior occipital gyrus; ITG, inferior temporal gyrus; MOG, middle occipital gyrus; MTG, middle temporal gyrus; ParOrb, pars orbitalis; ParsT, pars triangularis; ParsOp, pars opercularis; SLF, superior longitudinal fascicle; SMG, supramarginal gyrus; SOG, superior occipital gyrus; STG, superior temporal gyrus; VOF, vertical occipital fascicle).

in reply to sensory input. The frontal lobe constitutes, in fact, a collector of the different modalities of the language processing, and here the articulatory and motor planning for the final speech output occurs.

5.5.6 Language Planning and Output

Language planning and speech output are the result of a complex integration between hubs distributed between the posterior IFG and the VPMC, the IPL and the dorsal supplementary motor areas of the frontal lobe (in particular, SMA and pre-SMA), and the anterior third of the insula and the basal ganglia. These cortical and subcortical territories are interconnected by longitudinal associative bundles of the dorsal stream (in particular SLF III), transverse associative fibers (i.e., connecting dorsal and ventral cortices) of the frontal lobe (the so-called frontal aslant tract, FAT), projection fibers connecting dorsal and ventral premotor areas with basal ganglia, and even bi-hemispherical fibers of the anterior third of the corpus callosum.[31]

SAN is substantially subserved by POp, the ventral portions of the Pre-CG (i.e., VPMC) and Post-CG, and the IPL (i.e., SMG and AG). These areas are interconnected from a superficial layer of horizontal U-fibers and a deeper layer of long fibers (SLF III) essential for the motor-phonological planning and working memory. The stimulation of the VPMC, of the cortices of the IPL, and of the white matter underneath may elicit speech arrest (or verbal apraxia) regardless of the side of hemispherical specialization for language. SAN, in fact, is a network with a demonstrated bi-hemispherical organization.[32] This bilateral functional support is confirmed also by the recovery rate of face-mouth deficit and speech planning troubles after surgical resection, and evidences of a structural background of this bi-hemispheric organization were provided by high-resolution tractography and microdissection demonstrating homo- and heterotopic fibers connecting the VPMC of the two hemispheres and the VPMC of one hemisphere with the contralateral SMA.[31]

Finally, the motor control of language output is mediated by SMA (and pre-SMA) and the respective connectivity with the VPMC and basal ganglia provided, respectively, by the transverse fibers of the FAT and the fibers projecting from these premotor areas to caudate and putamen

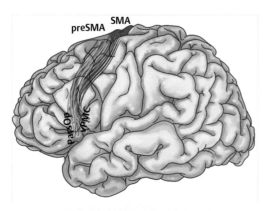

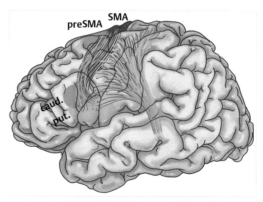

Fig. 5.24 Schematic representation of the transverse fibers of FAT connecting the dorsal supplementary motor areas with the ventral premotor cortex. (FAT, frontal aslant tract).

Fig. 5.25 Schematic representation of the projection fibers for language motor control (connecting the supplementary motor areas with the basal ganglia) and final output (ventral portion of the pyramidal tract) (Caud, caudate nucleus; Put, putamen; preSMA, pre-supplementary motor area; SMA, supplementary motor area).

(▶ Fig. 5.24 and ▶ Fig. 5.25).[33,34] The stimulation in this white matter area may produce speech arrest, especially in the most ventral portion, and speech arrest associated to motor movements arrest more dorsally, and perseverations.[8,9]

References

[1] Amunts K, Zilles K. Architectonic mapping of the human brain beyond Brodmann. Neuron. 2015; 88(6):1086–1107

[2] Tate MC, Herbet G, Moritz-Gasser S, Tate JE, Duffau H. Probabilistic map of critical functional regions of the human cerebral cortex: Broca's area revisited. Brain. 2014; 137(Pt 10):2773–2782

[3] Corina DP, Gibson EK, Martin R, Poliakov A, Brinkley J, Ojemann GA. Dissociation of action and object naming: evidence from cortical stimulation mapping. Hum Brain Mapp. 2005; 24(1):1–10

[4] Hickok G, Poeppel D. The cortical organization of speech processing. Nat Rev Neurosci. 2007; 8(5):393–402

[5] Makris N, Kennedy DN, McInerney S, et al. Segmentation of subcomponents within the superior longitudinal fascicle in humans: a quantitative, in vivo, DT-MRI study. Cereb Cortex. 2005; 15(6):854–869

[6] Wilson SM, Galantucci S, Tartaglia MC, et al. Syntactic processing depends on dorsal language tracts. Neuron. 2011; 72 (2):397–403

[7] Vigneau M, Beaucousin V, Hervé PY, et al. Meta-analyzing left hemisphere language areas: phonology, semantics, and sentence processing. Neuroimage. 2006; 30(4):1414–1432

[8] Sarubbo S, De Benedictis A, Merler S, et al. Towards a functional atlas of human white matter. Hum Brain Mapp. 2015; 36(8):3117–3136

[9] Sarubbo S, Tate M, De Benedictis A, et al. Mapping critical cortical hubs and white matter pathways by direct electrical stimulation: an original functional atlas of the human brain. Neuroimage. 2020; 205:116237

[10] Duffau H. Stimulation mapping of white matter tracts to study brain functional connectivity. Nat Rev Neurol. 2015; 11(5):255–265

[11] Duffau H, Moritz-Gasser S, Mandonnet E. A re-examination of neural basis of language processing: proposal of a dynamic hodotopical model from data provided by brain stimulation mapping during picture naming. Brain Lang. 2014; 131:1–10

[12] Duffau H, Taillandier L. New concepts in the management of diffuse low-grade glioma: proposal of a multistage and individualized therapeutic approach. Neuro-oncol. 2015; 17(3): 332–342

[13] Maffei C, Jovicich J, De Benedictis A, et al. Topography of the human acoustic radiation as revealed by ex vivo fibers micro-dissection and in vivo diffusion-based tractography. Brain Struct Funct. 2018; 223(1):449–459

[14] Maffei C, Sarubbo S, Jovicich J. A missing connection: a review of the macrostructural anatomy and tractography of the acoustic radiation. Front Neuroanat. 2019; 13:27

[15] Guenther FH, Hickok G. Role of the auditory system in speech production. In: Handbook of Clinical Neurology. 2015

[16] Sarubbo S, De Benedictis A, Milani P, et al. The course and the anatomo-functional relationships of the optic radiation: a combined study with "post mortem" dissections and "in vivo" direct electrical mapping. J Anat. 2015; 226(1):47–59

[17] De Benedictis A, Duffau H, Paradiso B, et al. Anatomo-functional study of the temporo-parieto-occipital region: dissection, tractographic and brain mapping evidence from a neurosurgical perspective. J Anat. 2014; 225(2):132–151

[18] Mandonnet E, Sarubbo S, Petit L. The Nomenclature of Human White Matter Association pathways: proposal for a systematic taxonomic anatomical classification. Front Neuroanat. 2018; 12:94

[19] Wang X, Pathak S, Stefaneanu L, Yeh FC, Li S, Fernandez-Miranda JC. Subcomponents and connectivity of the superior longitudinal fasciculus in the human brain. Brain Struct Funct. 2016; 221(4):2075–2092

[20] Thiebaut de Schotten M, Ffytche DH, Bizzi A, et al. Atlasing location, asymmetry and inter-subject variability of white matter tracts in the human brain with MR diffusion tractography. Neuroimage. 2011; 54(1):49–59

[21] Catani M, Jones DK, ffytche DH. Perisylvian language networks of the human brain. Ann Neurol. 2005; 57(1):8–16

[22] Sarubbo S, De Benedictis A, Merler S, et al. Structural and functional integration between dorsal and ventral language streams as revealed by blunt dissection and direct electrical stimulation. Hum Brain Mapp. 2016; 37(11):3858–3872

[23] Catani M, Jones DK, Donato R, Ffytche DH. Occipito-temporal connections in the human brain. Brain. 2003; 126 (Pt 9):2093–2107

[24] Zemmoura I, Herbet G, Moritz-Gasser S, Duffau H. New insights into the neural network mediating reading processes provided by cortico-subcortical electrical mapping. Hum Brain Mapp. 2015; 36(6):2215–2230

[25] Sarubbo S, De Benedictis A, Maldonado IL, Basso G, Duffau H. Frontal terminations for the inferior fronto-occipital fascicle: anatomical dissection, DTI study and functional considerations on a multi-component bundle. Brain Struct Funct. 2013; 218 (1):21–37

[26] Caverzasi E, Papinutto N, Amirbekian B, Berger MS, Henry RG. Q-ball of inferior fronto-occipital fasciculus and beyond. PLoS One. 2014; 9(6):e100274

[27] Hau J, Sarubbo S, Perchey G, et al. Cortical terminations of the inferior fronto-occipital and uncinate fasciculi: anatomical stem-based virtual dissection. Front Neuroanat. 2016; 10:58

[28] Herbet G, Moritz-Gasser S, Duffau H. Direct evidence for the contributive role of the right inferior fronto-occipital fasciculus in non-verbal semantic cognition. Brain Struct Funct. 2017; 222(4):1597–1610

[29] Hau J, Sarubbo S, Houde JC, et al. Revisiting the human uncinate fasciculus, its subcomponents and asymmetries with stem-based tractography and microdissection validation. Brain Struct Funct. 2017; 222(4):1645–1662

[30] Papagno C, Casarotti A, Comi A, et al. Long-term proper name anomia after removal of the uncinate fasciculus. Brain Struct Funct. 2016; 221(1):687–694

[31] De Benedictis A, Petit L, Descoteaux M, et al. New insights in the homotopic and heterotopic connectivity of the frontal portion of the human corpus callosum revealed by microdissection and diffusion tractography. Hum Brain Mapp. 2016; 37(12):4718–4735

[32] Zacà D, Corsini F, Rozzanigo U, et al. Whole-brain network connectivity underlying the human speech articulation as emerged integrating direct electric stimulation, resting state fMRI and tractography. Front Hum Neurosci. 2018; 12:405

[33] Catani M, Mesulam MM, Jakobsen E, et al. A novel frontal pathway underlies verbal fluency in primary progressive aphasia. Brain. 2013; 136(Pt 8):2619–2628

[34] Catani M, Dell'acqua F, Vergani F, et al. Short frontal lobe connections of the human brain. Cortex. 2012; 48(2):273–291

6 What You Need to Know About Electricity

6.1 The Scope of This Chapter

IONM is about detection, interpretation, and manipulation of bioelectricity in the nervous system (and muscle tissue). Before we address the technical methods to monitor and interact with brain functions, we will review the basic concepts of "electricity" and how electricity interferes with the brain. If you work with or at least want to understand neurophysiological monitoring you need to be familiar with some physics. On the other hand, if you are eager for the practical applications, skip this chapter and come back later.

6.2 Basics of Electricity—Some Useful Definitions

6.2.1 Voltage (V), Potential (P), Current (I), Resistance (Ω), Power (W), and Frequency (Hz)

The part of an atom that gives an element the identity is the nucleus. The nucleus is made of protons (positively charged) and neutrons (neutral). Negatively charged electrons surround the nucleus. If the number of electrons does not equal the number of protons, the atom or molecule becomes an ion.

An atom with less electrons is positively charged (cation). An atom with more electrons is negatively charged (anion). Same charges repulse, and unlike charges attract each other (▶ Fig. 6.1).

Conductors are atoms that can pass electrons (i.e., charges can move freely, e.g., copper).

Insulators are atoms with no free electrons; hence, the charge is not easily transported (e.g., rubber).

Electrons in a conductor move freely from atom to atom in a completely random way. The force to get them moving in a determined direction is the *electromotive force* (*EMF*, or simply *E*), commonly known as **voltage**. Voltage is a difference in charge between two points.

Connecting these points with a conductor will induce the flow of electrons (*current*) from negatively charged atoms to positively charged atoms. This current continues until an equilibrium is reached and both sides of the circuit become electrically neutral.

A difference in charge induces a potential flow (current) of electrons between the different charged positions, therefore the term **potential**.

The unit which measures voltage is volt (**V**). Voltages can be (according to the point of reference) positive or negative. In a battery, the voltage at the positive terminal is +1.5 V relative to the negative

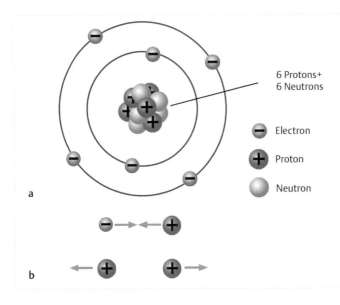

6 Protons+
6 Neutrons

Electron

Proton

Neutron

a

b

Fig. 6.1 (a) Simple model of the carbon atom, demonstrating the concept of positive and negative charges. **(b)** Same charges repulse, and unlike charges attract each other.

terminal. The voltage at the negative terminal is −1.5 V relative to the positive terminal. Current flow is directly proportional to the potential difference between these two points (Ohm's law).

Current is measured in **ampere (I)**. Ampere describes the number of electrons passing through a cross-section of a conductor per second. The higher the number of amperes the higher the number of electrons that pass through a cross-section of the conductor per second.

This flow is dependent on the electrical resistance of the conductor: current flow is inversely correlated to the resistance of the conductor. The unit of resistance is **Ohm (R)**.

Ohm's law: Current flow through a conductor (wire) between two points is directly proportional to the potential difference across the two points, and inversely proportional to the resistance between them.

$$V = RI.$$

Example: When 1 Volt is placed across 1 ohm of resistance, there will be a current of 1 Ampere.

Electric power is the work performed. Power is measured in watts (**P**). The term *Wattage* is commonly used for "electric power in watts." One watt is the rate at which electrical work is performed when a current of one ampere (A) flows across an electrical potential difference of one volt (V).

$$P = VI$$

Current is the flow of electrons, measured in Ampere, past a point in a circuit in a defined amount of time. 1 A = 1 Coulomb (= 6,242,000,000,000,000 electrons/sec). As electrons are negatively charged, they flow from negative terminal to the positive terminal.

There are two main types of current flow: "Direct Current (DC) and Alternating Current (AC)."

Basically, in DC, the "direction" of current flow remains constant over time, whereas, in AC, the direction of flow of current keeps alternating from one direction to the other. The number of changes in direction, the *frequency* is measured in Hertz (Hz). 1 Hertz is one change per second. In the United States, alternating current changes 60 times a second (60 Hz). In the Europe it happens at 50 Hz (60 Hz Stimulator/50 Hz Stimulator). By the way, AC is more dangerous than DC as it can cause ventricular fibrillations at a much lower current as DC.

6.2.2 How to Measure Electricity

An *Ohmmeter* is an instrument which measures the electrical resistance.

A *Voltmeter* measures the electrical potential difference between two points in an electrical circuit.

An *Ammeter* measures the electric current in a circuit.

6.3 The Electric Fields

An electric field is a vector field. This field is caused by an electric charge that applies forces on other charges, attracting (different charges) or repelling them (same charges). In this vector field each point is characterized by a force, called the Coulomb force. The units of the electric field in the SI system are newtons per coulomb (N/C), or volts per meter (V/m). The electric field and the magnetic field together form the electromagnetic force, one of the four fundamental forces of nature (▶ Fig. 6.2).

Clinical application: The geometric configuration of the electric field induced by opposite charges is very important for the bioelectric stimulation and detection of bioelectricity of the CNS. The understanding of electric fields is fundamental for understanding how IONM works. You will see this in the following chapters.

6.4 The Electricity of the Nervous System

The major functions of the nervous system are depending on the generation, conduction, and integration of electrical activity in combination with the synthesis and release of neurotransmitter.

Nervous system electricity as a correlate to nervous system activity and functionality is thus present in neurons and axons.

- IONM is *monitoring* these electrical activities.
- IONM is *interfering* with these processes.

In the following we will therefore review "the electricity of the brain."

6.4.1 The Action Potential

Here we explain the fundamental principle of signal generation on the level of the cell membrane. As this is a fundamental mechanism which constitutes the basis of detecting and manipulating the "electricity of the brain" we need to go a little more into details.

The membranes of neurons and axons are electrically **polarized.** In the resting state the outside is positively charged and the inside negatively. The

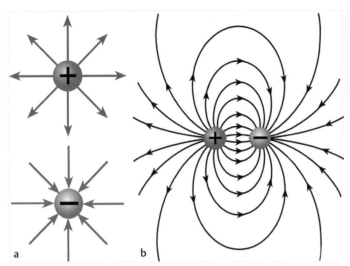

Fig. 6.2 (a) An electric field is caused by an electric charge that applies forces on other charges, attracting (different charges) or repelling them (same charges). **(b)** In this vector field, each point is characterized by a force, called the Coulomb force.

a   b

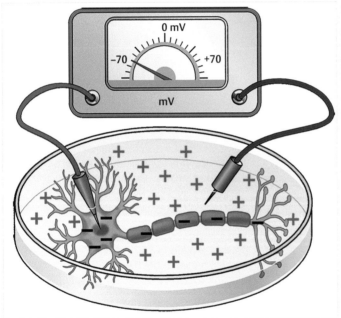

Fig. 6.3 The membranes of neurons and axons are electrically polarized. The resting membrane potential is around −70 mV.

difference in **voltage** between the inside of the cell and its exterior environment in the not activated cell is called **resting membrane potential**. The default voltage is around −70 mV (▸ Fig. 6.3). As long as the neuron isn't "firing" it maintains this resting potential by moving **ions** (positively or negatively charged atoms) in and out of itself (▸ Fig. 6.4).

If at the outside of the membrane (neuron or axon) the charge changes at a certain threshold (−50 mV) the permeability of the membrane is changed and voltage-gated **sodium** ion channels open and shift the membrane potential to more positive potential inside the membrane: a **depolarization** of the membrane occurs (▸ Fig. 6.5). This is an *all or none response.* If the membrane potential reaches +30 mV the sodium channel closes (▸ Fig. 6.6). At this point the membrane has changed charge: the outside is negatively charged and the inside positively. Now voltage-gated **potassium** channels open and positively charged

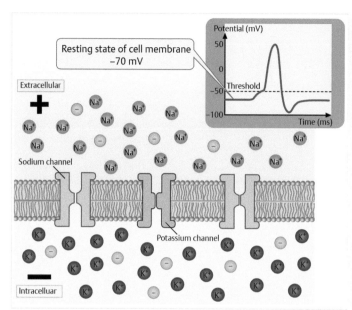

Fig. 6.4 The cell maintains the resting potential of −70 mV by moving ions (positively or negatively charged atoms) in and out of itself.

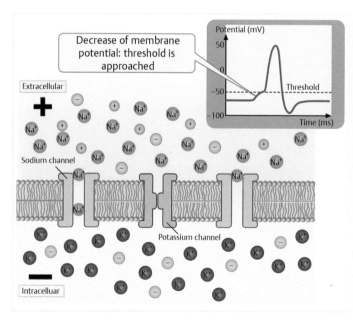

Fig. 6.5 If the charge changes at a certain threshold (−50 mV), the permeability of the membrane is changed and voltage-gated **sodium** ion channels open: a **depolarization** of the membrane occurs.

K⁺ ions rush to the outside of the membrane, resulting in a **repolarization** of the membrane (▶ Fig. 6.7). As the potassium channels close with a little delay, a **hyperpolarization** occurs. Until the deactivated sodium channels become reactivated, the membrane is refractory for the next depolarization: the "refractory period." Eventually, adenosine triphosphate-dependent ion pump transports sodium to the outside of the membrane and potassium to the inside: the membrane returns to the resting state and can be depolarized again. This takes only around 4.4 ms, so the membrane can be depolarized for several hundred times in a second.

As an action potential (nerve impulse) travels down an axon, there is a change in polarity across the membrane of the axon. The impulse moves

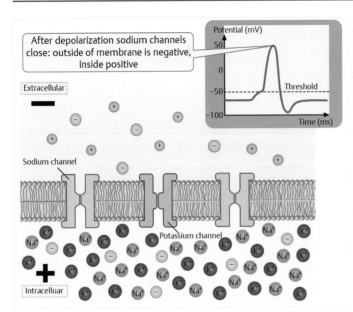

Fig. 6.6 After depolarization the membrane has changed charge: the outside is negatively and the inside is positively charged.

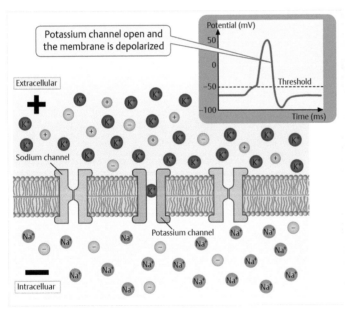

Fig. 6.7 Positively charged K⁺ ions rush to the outside of the membrane, resulting in a repolarization of the membrane.

down the axon, toward the axon terminal. This occurs in one direction only (▶ Fig. 6.8). At the axon terminal, a transfer of the signal via the synapses occurs.

This is all **simplified**, just to explain the principle. In reality, neuron membranes incorporate several **types** of ion pumps and channels, which can be **gated** by all sorts of **triggers** besides just voltage; and their firing **patterns** are much more complex. Read up on it, but keep it simple in your mind.

Now we need to understand how this principle applies to the communication between neurons.

6.4.2 Postsynaptic Potentials

When the action potential reaches the terminal, its wave of depolarization opens voltage-activated

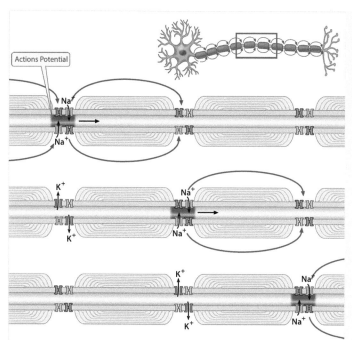

Actions Potential

Na⁺

Na⁺

K⁺

K⁺

Na⁺

Na⁺

K⁺

K⁺

Na⁺

Na⁺

Fig. 6.8 The action potential travels down the axon. There is a change in polarity across the membrane of the axon. The impulse moves down the axon, toward the axon terminal. This occurs in one direction only.

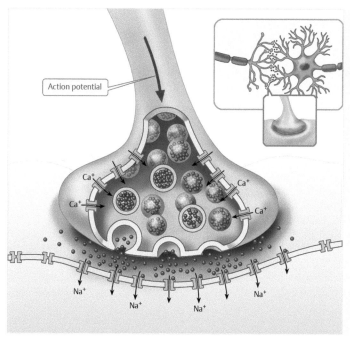

Action potential

Ca⁺

Ca⁺

Ca⁺

Ca⁺

Na⁺

Na⁺

Na⁺

Na⁺

Fig. 6.9 When the action potential reaches the terminal its wave of depolarization opens voltage-activated Ca^{2+} channels and neurotransmitters are released across synaptic gap.

Ca^{2+} channels (▶ Fig. 6.9). Ca^{2+} induces vesicles to fuse with presynaptic cell membrane. Neurotransmitters are released across synaptic gap. The binding of neurotransmitter to receptors on the postsynaptic cell of the next cells dendrites changes the permeability of the cell membrane and therefore the net charge of the postsynaptic neuron. A postsynaptic potential is induced. As multiple axons

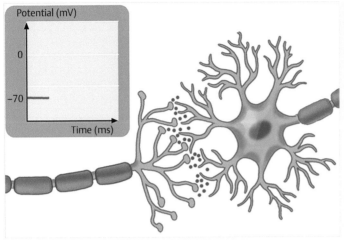

Fig. 6.10 A postsynaptic potential is induced. As multiple axons reach multiple dendrites this does not happen as a single event.

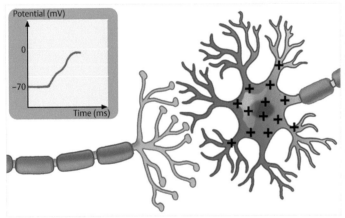

Fig. 6.11 An excitatory postsynaptic potentials (EPSPs) cause ions to flow into the cell and depolarize the cell.

reach multiple dendrites this does not happen as a single event (▶ Fig. 6.10). Unlike action potential, which can only be excitatory, postsynaptic potentials can be excitatory or inhibitory. Excitatory Postsynaptic Potentials (EPSP) cause ions to flow into the cell and depolarize the cell (▶ Fig. 6.11). Inhibitory postsynaptic potentials (IPSPs) make postsynaptic membrane more negative as ions flow out of the cell (▶ Fig. 6.12). The way a neuron's EPSPs and IPSPs summate to cause or prevent a spike correlates to the sum of multiple events. Postsynaptic potentials are therefore graded responses; they can vary in amplitude and they last much longer than action potentials.

Clinical application: As we will see later, what EEG and SSEP are actually recording is the sum *of Postsynaptic Potentials happening in a large number of events. They can be detected because they are occurring slowly (as compared to AP) at the same time or at the same location.*

6.4.3 Induction of Muscle Action

If neurons involved in motor areas are stimulated, these activities will eventually induce muscle actions. Let us have a short look into this mechanism.

A volley of electrical activity travels along the corticospinal tract, interfering with the motor unit. A motor unit is made up of a motor neuron and the skeletal muscle fibers innervated by that motor neuron's axonal terminal. The axon of a motor neuron terminates on the muscle fiber:

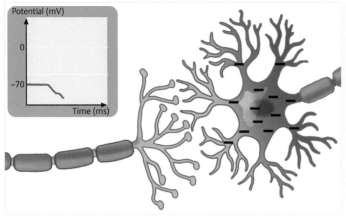

Fig. 6.12 Inhibitory postsynaptic potentials (IPSPs) make postsynaptic membrane more negative as ions flow out of the cell.

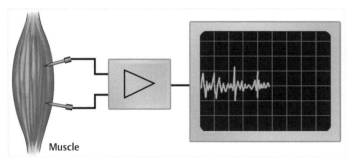

Fig. 6.13 The principle of recording compound muscle action potentials (CMAPs) by using pairs of surface or needle electrodes that are placed into the belly of a muscle.

the neuromuscular junction. If the action potential reaches the chemical synapse, it releases a neurotransmitter (acetylcholine). This transmitter binds to the acetylcholine receptor, a protein in the membrane of the muscle fiber and triggers the action potential of the muscle.

The muscle action potential lasts around 2 to 4 ms, the absolute refractory period is roughly 1 to 3 ms. The action potential releases calcium ions that free up the tropomyosin and allow the muscle to contract.

6.4.4 Compound Muscle Activity

The responses that are elicited are summed responses from many muscle fibers known as compound muscle action potentials (CMAPs). They can be recorded using pairs of surface or needle electrodes that are placed over or into the belly of a muscle (▶ Fig. 6.13).

These are in a simplified way the principles of bioelectricity in the CNS. Let us now investigate how to detect these activities.

6.5 Detect the Electricity of the Nervous System

IONM detects the electrical activity due to changes in membrane voltage at the level of the effector organ, i.e., the muscle, at the cortical level (i.e., motor cortex, somatosensory cortex), and at the axonal level (white matter fiber tracts, brainstem, spinal cord). The substrate that IONM measures is the difference in voltage (potential) between two electrodes. This can, for research applications, be done for the single neuron and axon. IONM, however, evaluates the summation of potentials that are generated by whole swathes of tissue that contain millions of neurons, axons, and muscle fibers.

As single neuron axon or muscle fiber produces very weak fields, *IONM recordings are only possible for events that are spatiotemporally coherent and locally synchronized.*

What IONM is therefore actually recording is the sum of events. This is the postsynaptic potential (PSP), more precisely the temporal (PSPs occurred close in time, i.e., triggered by a stimulation) or the spatial summation (PSPs occur in close proximity: detection of cortical activity somatosensory cortex).

In other words, IONM detects responses of the NS on stimuli or events (event-related potentials, **ERP**). For example, the cortical activity triggered by the stimulation of a peripheral nerve can be detected with the technique of SSEPs or somewhat vice versa the CMAPs triggered by cortical stimulation of motor cortex: motor-evoked potentials (MEPs).

In the following we will explain the electrophysiological principles of recording changes in membrane voltage fundamental principles that you need to understand EEGs, SSEPs, and MEPs. A very important concept is the dipole.

6.5.1 The Dipole

The dipole is simply a separation of unlike charges over distance (▶ Fig. 6.2). The concept of the dipole is fundamental for the detecting and measuring of EEG and SSEP.

Let us have a look at postsynaptic potentials again.

An excitatory postsynaptic potential (EPSP) is caused by the influx of positive ions into the cell body of the neuron, inducing a positive charge of the neuron (▶ Fig. 6.11). In contrast, an inhibitory postsynaptic potential (IPSP) hyperpolarizes the cell membrane by making the membrane potential more negative (▶ Fig. 6.12). EPSP and IPSP form a separation of charge and thus form a dipole.

If in the pyramidal cells of the cortex an EPSP induces an influx of positive charges into the cell, the intracellular space will become more positive and thus the extracellular space relatively more negative. As this typically occurs near the cell body, the apical dendrite (typical for pyramidal cells) will become relatively more positive than the extracellular space at the reception site (▶ Fig. 6.14).

This separation of unlike charges over distance forms a dipole. The current flows from the positive site (source) to the negative site (sink). An IPSP also forms a dipole, only with the reverse polarity (▶ Fig. 6.15).

The individual potential created by the cellular dipoles is too weak to be detected. However, the summation of "bipolar" activity of several thousands of neurons (▶ Fig. 6.16) can be detected by a Voltmeter. As we are measuring very small electrical activities, we need a very sensitive voltmeter (bioamplifier).

The summation depends on two factors:
1. The timing of the neural activity. When neurons fire at different times, the signal will be too

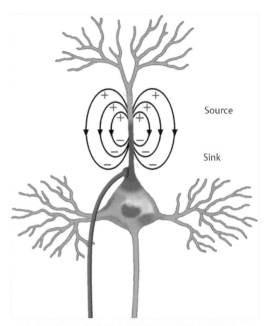

Fig. 6.14 Excitatory postsynaptic potential (EPSP) triggers influx of positive charges into the cell. Ultimately a polarization at the apical dendrite will be induced. This separation of unlike charges over distance forms a dipole.

weak to be detected. If they fire at the same time, however, the signal might become strong enough to be detected.
2. The orientation of the neurons (dipoles). If the neurons (dipoles) are in opposite alignment, the dipoles will neutralize each other and the signal will not be detected. If they are scattered, only a weak signal will be detected. The strongest signal will be generated if the neurons are aligned toward the sensors or (and that has huge practical applications) the sensor is aligned toward the neurons.

Clinical application: These phenomena explain why we can only detect synchronized activity (i.e., SSEPs) or clusters of activities (i.e., EEG/ECoG).

6.5.2 The Electrical Field of a Dipole

The separation of unlike charges over distance (definition of a dipole) induces a field in which repulsive and attracting forces are combined in a three-dimensional space. The properties of the electric field at any given point are dependent on the summation of the attracting and repulsive forces that are induced by the positive and negative charges.

This electrical charge can be determined by vector addition.

If we consider an isolated charge the force of it on any given point is dependent on the distance (inverse square law). The direction of the force will be oriented toward the source (negative charged source) or away (positive charged source) (▶ Fig. 6.1 and ▶ Fig. 6.2). If we now look at the force that is exerted in a dipole, the electrical field at any given point is the summation of the attracting and repulsive forces.

Clinical application: This concept is especially important to understand the electrical force that

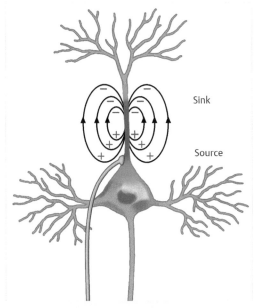

Fig. 6.15 An inhibitory postsynaptic potential (IPSP) also forms a dipole, only with the reverse polarity.

we apply be using anodal/cathodal or cathodal/anodal stimulation (monopolar stimulation). It also explains why SSEP signals are so susceptible to changes of the brains position. If the distance changes (i.e., positioning, insertion of a spreader) due to the inverse square law, changes in configuration of the detected signal can be substantial (▶ Fig. 6.17).

Another major problem in measuring the potential differences in the CNS arises from the fact that we are not measuring electricity in a simple, linear conductor (i.e., copper wire), but in a very inhomogeneous matrix: nerves, muscles, and the brain. Different tissues with different impedances are not in linear alignment, but in a three-dimensional, inhomogeneous system.

Clinical application: If you think about the manipulation of the tissue during surgery (irrigation, blood clots, cottonoids, temperature changes, etc.) you will appreciate that IONM is a very dynamic process.

So, IONM measures a very tiny potential difference in a complex volume with dynamic changes regarding position and impedance.

In the following we want to provide the basis for understanding the way in which bioelectric currents are conducted in tissues and how this determines the detection of the potentials recorded.

An obvious problem is that the amplitude that you measure at your recording electrode is inversely correlated with the distance from the source (distance square law). The equation for this is:

$$v = \frac{q}{4\pi E_0 r}$$

v = q (Charge at the source)/$4\pi\, E_0$ (which is a constant), r (= radius) (▶ Fig. 6.17).

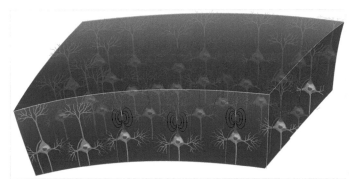

Fig. 6.16 The individual potential created by the cellular dipoles is too weak to be detected. However, the summation of "bipolar" activity of several thousands of neurons can be detected by a Voltmeter.

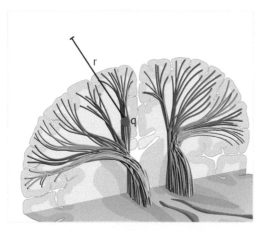

Fig. 6.17 The amplitude of the signal is inversely correlated with the distance from the source.

6.5.3 Volume Conduction: Detecting Dipoles

The term "volume conduction" refers to the complex effects of detecting and measuring (or applying) electrical potentials at a distance from the current source (the place where the potential is actually happening), in a three-dimensional space. Volume conduction is an essential concept, in particular, all clinical neurophysiological recordings, both central and peripheral, since recording electrodes cannot be placed in direct contact with the tissue generating the signal. In fact, volume conductive effects substantially impact all motor and sensory nerve conduction waveforms. The characteristics of SSEP, EEG, and MEP recordings are correlated with volume conductive effects.

There are two basic types of current sources to consider:

1. **Moving sources** are dipoles formed by action potentials that move, either along nerve or muscle fibers. Thus, the action potentials are active areas, which move along the fiber structures. Other parts of the structure remain electrically silent. Examples: nerve action potentials or electromyographic (EMG) potentials.
2. **Stationary sources**: Dipoles formed by action potentials that arise from nonmoving sources such as nerve cell bodies or their dendrites. Clinical important examples: SSEPs and EEG. These are also referred to as field, or sink/source potentials.

For the measuring of bioelectricity in a volume, two additional concepts need to be introduced: Solid angles and summation of solid angles.

6.5.4 Solid Angles

The recording electrode on the surface of the skull (be it for EEG or SSEEP) measures a bipolar potential in a three-dimensional object: a volume. Imagine that the electrode "sees" the volume from a distance. The size and configuration of the object depend on the angle from which the observer watches. In geometry this is quantified by the concept of a **solid angle** (symbol: Ω). The concept of solid angle explains why the position of the electrode or the angle of the recording electrode toward the source is of great importance. Ω is a measure of the amount of the field of view from some particular point that a given object covers. That is, it is a measure of how large the object appears to an observer looking from that point. The physical properties of this concept are complicated; nevertheless, these are important to understand fundamental principles in IONM: As the change of the angle is directly proportional to the amplitude of the signal you are measuring, the relative position of electrodes which measure the signal in relation to the signal is of utmost importance.

Clinical application: The important practical application of this complicated topic lies in the fact that if the position of the electrodes (i.e., scalp electrodes) changes (i.e., putting in a spreader) or position of the signal generator (cortical areas of brain) changes (resection-induced brain shift) your recorded signal might change dramatically (▶ Fig. 7.5a, b).

If the position of the recording electrode is changed, this will result in marked changes in the solid angle, even though the event itself remains unchanged.

Or, if the source is moving and the recording electrode is stationary the relative solid angle electrode positions below the level of the interface will result in apparent reversal of polarity, even though the event itself remains unchanged.

In brain tumor surgery, with the very dynamic positional changes of the structures of interest you need to prepare for the right interpretation of these changes, as we will explain in the following chapters.

As we have now laid the groundwork to understand the "bioelectricity of the brain" we can now discuss the practical applications most relevant to IONM.

7 Transcranial Monitoring—Methods to Monitor CNS Functions: Principles

7.1 The Scope of This Chapter

We will first introduce the principles of EEG, SSEP, and MEP monitoring in the transcranial setting. In the second part of this section we will look at the direct cortical or subcortical applications of these techniques.

7.2 EEG

In a nutshell, electroencephalography is a principal technique in neuroscience to study basic features of sleep, coma, epilepsy, and brain death. EEG studies the spontaneous (in opposite to SSEPs) electrical activity of the brain. For IONM this technique is of particular interest as intraoperative electrocorticography (ECoG) is an import adjunct to direct cortical and subcortical stimulation.

EEG measures the potentials that are induced by the summated activity of EPSPs and IPSPs at the dendritic synapses of the pyramidal cells (▶ Fig. 6.14 and ▶ Fig. 6.15) that are found in the fifth layer of the cerebral cortex. The waves in the EEG reflect voltage fluctuations caused by thousands of neurons. EPSPs and IPSPs cause dipoles, which are the "substrates" of the EEG recording. The orientation of the dipole is important for the detection and quantification. Dipole orientation is correlated with the orientation of the cells and can be radial (vertical) or horizontal (tangential) and anything between.

In summary, the dipole's potential varies inversely with the square of the distance from the source (distance square law) and depends on the angle from the dipole's axis (solid angle). This has important practical applications: the position of the dipole is directly correlated with a decrease or increase or orientation of the detected amplitude. Though EEG also detects the amplitude of the microcurrent, the major feature of interest is the frequency of the generation of the dipoles as surrogate parameter of the metabolic activity near the recording electrodes. In contrast to SSEP, which are very small dipoles also induced by action potentials and often do not exceed 3 µV in size, EEG potentials are in the range of 10 to 50 µV and last 10 to 250 ms (as compared to 1–2 ms for action potentials).

Anesthesia with inhalation agents has a profound effect on EEG with associated decreased excitation up to burst suppression and isoelectricity. As IONM works with total intravenous anesthesia (TIVA) only, we will not go through EEG changes induced by inhalation agents. Note, however, that TIVA also induces some changes in the EEG pattern.

7.2.1 How EEG Works—Principles

The standard EEG recording uses 21 head leads with an impedance between 100 and 5000 Ω.

Frequencies that are filtered out are those below 0.3 t 1 Hz (low pass) and above 35 t 70 Hz.

The recording electrodes are arranged following the International 10–20 System (▶ Fig. 7.1).

In principle, you need to measure the distance between the nasion and the inion in the sagittal plane (midline above the sinus) and do the same in the axial plane. The position of the electrodes is defined by the cross-section of either the 10 or 20% longitude or latitude lines.

Explanation of the nomenclature: F(Frontal), Fp (Frontopolar), T(Temporal), C(Central), P(Parietal), O(Occipital). The letter A stands for the lobules of the ear. Pg stands for nasopharyngeal and Fp for frontal polar sites. Z stands for "zero line" which is the midline in the sagittal plane (following the sagittal sinus). Additional odd number identifies the left side, even number the right side.

The signal measured by one electrode must be referred to a similar electrode (theoretically inactive) for all electrodes (referential montage) or to another active electrode (bipolar montage). Referential is used in the diagnostic labs, bipolar in the OR.

The frequency of the recorded signals is one of the fundamental features of the EEG (▶ Fig. 7.2).

Mnemo: DTAB delta <4, and theta ≥4, and <8, and alpha ≥8, and <14, and Beta ≥14.

In the OR settings, the frequencies are analyzed by observation: "eyeballing." That means: "count" the waves in a one-second interval. The more intense the cortical activity, the smaller the amplitude and the higher the frequency; less intense cortical activity leads to slower waves with larger amplitude.

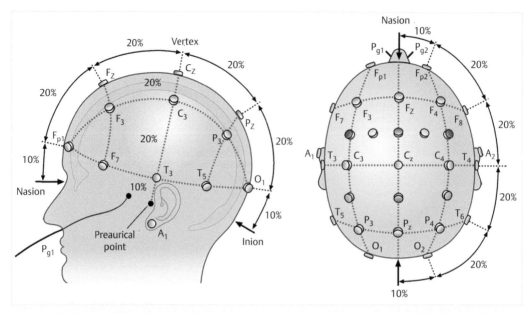

Fig. 7.1 The International 10–20 system.

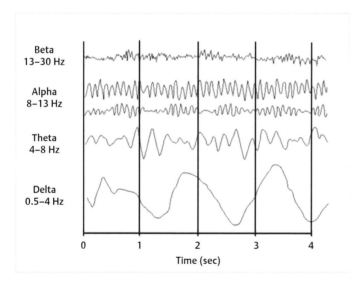

Fig. 7.2 The frequency of the electroencephalography (EEG) with nomenclature. Mnemo: DTAB, delta <4, and theta ≥4, and <8, and alpha ≥8, and <14, and beta ≥14.

The EEG patterns that are recorded when a patient transits from an awake thought process to deep sleep is very similar compared to the induction of anesthesia. The typical difference between awake and anesthetized patient is the transition from beta waves (awake) to alpha waves (anesthetized). For the awake patient (for us of interest during awake craniotomies), the EEG will show high-frequency, low-amplitude beta waves, which is helpful when waiting for the extubation in an asleep/awake setting. In the awake patient EMG artifact is obvious, mostly from facial and ocular muscles. These are characterized by high-amplitude and high-frequency activity. Blinks, for example, are represented by sharp deflections.

Intraoperative EEG monitoring (ECoG) is very useful for detection of seizures, which are usually detected as spikes or wave complexes (▶ Fig. 7.3).

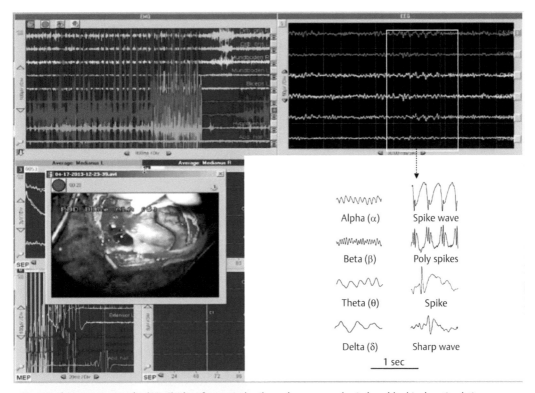

Fig. 7.3 Electrocorticography (ECoG) identifies typical spike and wave complex induced by bipolar stimulation.

7.3 SSEP

In a nutshell, SSEP provides you with information about the functionality of the somatosensory system. By stimulation of a peripheral nerve (i.e., the median or tibial nerve) a signal volley (membrane potential) is induced, which travels through the peripheral nerve, plexus, spinal column, brainstem, thalamus until it reaches the cortical surface. This signal can be filtered from the background noise since the stimulation time is known (time resolution) and the technique uses a high repetition rate. The stimulus can be detected at multiple anatomical levels: here we will focus on the detection and interpretation of the signal at the cortical level. The signal is analyzed regarding the time needed from stimulus generation to detection (latency) and morphology/size of the signal (amplitude) (▶ Fig. 7.4).

The point of interest of SSEPs in the context of surgical IONM is mainly the fact that SSEPs provide you with a global, quite sensitive warning system.

In principle, SSEPs are sequentially recorded and compared: initially before surgery starts (baselines) with further check-up recordings in due

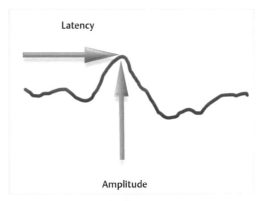

Fig. 7.4 Evaluation of the somatosensory-evoked potential (SSEP) signal: the time needed from stimulus generation to detection (latency) and morphology/size of the signal (amplitude).

course. As we have pointed out in the previous chapter, the recording of the SSEPs is highly dependent on the position of the detecting electrodes in relation to the source. Obviously, these positions are not fixed: during a dynamic surgical

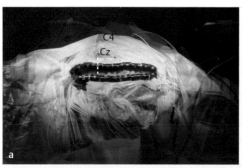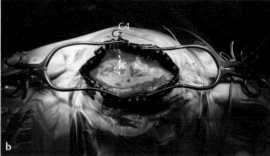

Fig. 7.5 **(a)** Position of Cz and C4 before insertion of the spreader. **(b)** Position of Cz and C4 after insertion of the spreader: relative position to the midline plus 2 cm: Cz is now in position of C4.

procedure these electrodes are displaced in their position (▶ Fig. 7.4a, b) or the source is displaced (brain shift). In consequence, amplitude of signals is variable (latency much more robust) and several baseline investigations are necessary to adapt to different stages of resection.

Again, SSEPs present an average of responses which are recorded after many repetitive stimulations. The initial recordings are called baseline and are the reference.

It needs hundreds of stimuli to record a well-formed, reliable SSEP (▶ **Video 7.1**). As repetitive trials are needed to establish a sufficient average, it can take seconds to minutes to record an SSEP. Thus, the response is always delayed and is never a "live" indicator of neuronal functions.

Changes in the SSEP may correspond to evolving injury somewhere along the pathway between stimulating and recording electrodes. In order to detect changes in SSEPs, the responses must be quantified. Thus, when we record SSEPs, we look at the following variable parameters (▶ Fig. 7.4):

Latency: Nerve conduction times are well defined. If we stimulate a nerve at the wrist, we know that it takes approximately 9 ms for that activity to reach the shoulder, 13 ms to reach the cervical spine, and 20 ms to reach the cerebral cortex. Thus, if we record at those points, we should expect to see responses at 9, 13, and 20 ms after stimulus onset, with individual variability. Conduction time is however susceptible to low temperatures, blood pressure, and depth of the anesthesia. If you can rule these effects out, increases in these latencies can be indicative of evolving injury.

Amplitude: SSEP amplitude varies by recording location and patient (individual variability,

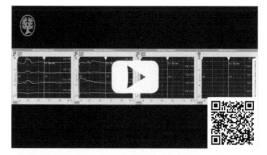

Video 7.1 Typical SSEP baseline.

pathology, etc.). So, only a substantial decrease in amplitude *in relation* to baseline recordings can be indicative of evolving injury.

As long as SSEPs are ok, a large part of the CNS (the somatosensory system) is ok. Subtle changes might predict pending disaster, might induce counter reactions, or might even indicate a termination of the procedure. Therefore, it is mandatory that you have a principal knowledge of how SSEPs work and probably more important: what are the limitations of this method.

What is the SSEP recording?

The source of SSEPs is the synaptic activity of sensory neurons (thalamus, somatosensory cortex) and the action potential along axons (i.e., brachial plexus). SSEP monitors therefore stationary sources and traveling sources. As compared to the EEG signal, the recorded signals are very small. They can be recorded nevertheless, because the signal that we want to detect within the "noise" is directly correlated to a stimulus that is applied, controlled, and therefore precisely known. After a high number of stimuli (around 500) an average is made. As the background noise is cancelling itself by its random appearance and not correlated to the stimulus, the signal remains. This is the principle how evoked potential works (▶ **Video 7.1**).

7.3.1 Correlation Between SSEPs and Cerebral Perfusion

Clinical application: Similar to the EEG recording, there is an almost linear correlation between cerebral blood flow and SSEP amplitude. This makes SSEP recording very important for the early detection of vascular problems, especially important in surgery in which lenticular-striatal arteries are involved.

7.3.2 How SSEP Works—Principles

SSEP works with the application of a stimulus to a nerve and the detection of the induced electrical volley as it runs through the somatosensory nervous system (▶ Fig. 5.8).

How Can a Nerve be Stimulated?

We need to induce an action potential at the membrane of the nerve. The principle of the action potential has been explained in chapter "The electricity of the Nervous System." Let us now look into the details we need to understand for the application of a stimulus to a membrane of a neuron or nerve (we will simplify to get the concept). To induce a membrane potential, we need to apply a potential to the membrane that is overcoming the threshold of the membrane. To this end we need a neurostimulator.

How Does a Neurostimulator Work?

It applies current to biological tissue. We will explain the principles here, but for a deeper understanding of this important concept we recommend to read in more depth.[1] The settings of the stimulator determine whether anions (−) and cations (+) are applied. The cathode of the neurostimulator is the negative pole (−) because it applies anions (−), and the anode is the positive pole (+) because it applies cations (+). Therefore, cathodal stimulation discharges anions (−) as current flows from the cathode (−), through the tissue, and back to the anode (+). In anodal stimulation, cations (+) are discharged into the body as current flows from the anode (+), through the tissue, and back to the cathode (−) (▶ Fig. 7.6).

Let us place an electrical stimulator near the tibial nerve (▶ Fig. 7.7). If we start cathodal stimulation a flow of negatively charged anions (−) is induced. They flow from the cathode, into the tissue, and back to the anode. As the electrical current flows from cathode to anode, negative charges accumulate on the outer nerve membrane. This makes the outside of the membrane more negative. Consequently, the inside of the membrane becomes more positive due to the attraction of positive ions. This will eventually result in depolarization and, if the threshold is reached, this will result in an action potential (nerve impulse or muscle activation)

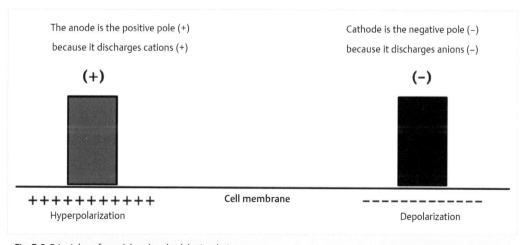

The anode is the positive pole (+)

because it discharges cations (+)

(+)

+++++++++++   Cell membrane

Hyperpolarization

Cathode is the negative pole (−)

because it discharges anions (−)

(−)

−−−−−−−−−−−−−

Depolarization

Fig. 7.6 Principles of anodal and cathodal stimulation.

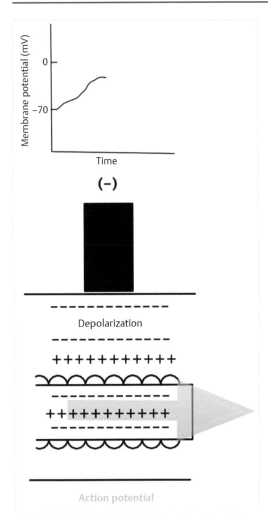

Fig. 7.7 Cathodal stimulation induces a flow of negatively charged anions (−). This makes the outside of the membrane more negative and will eventually result in depolarization and, if the threshold is reached, result in an action potential (nerve impulse or muscle activation).

(▶ Fig. 6.4 and ▶ Fig. 6.7). As a result of stimulation, an action potential is sent in both directions along the length of the nerve. As at the anode negative charges are attracted, the outer membrane of the cell becomes electrically positive as compared to the inner membrane. The cell is **hyperpolarized** under the anode, meaning that it is difficult to activate. This is called anodal block (▶ Fig. 7.8). To avoid an anodal block by stimulation of a nerve the **anode should be placed distally**, and the **cathode should be placed proximally**.

After the induction of an AP, the AP will be conducted down the membrane. As the membrane needs some time before depolarization can occur again (restitution of the electrochemical gradient), the AP can only run into one direction (that is preventing that an AP bounces back and forth) and the induction of the next AP will take some time: that is the refractory time. There is an absolute refractory time: Na$^+$ gates are closed and inactivated, no action potential can occur. In the relative refractory period an action potential can occur, but the stimulus must be much larger to overcome the relative refractory period. And the stimulus must not hit the membrane in the absolute refractory period (around 4 ms *interstimulus interval* (▶ Fig. 6.4 and ▶ Fig. 6.7). So, if we sustain a threshold stimulus, the absolute refractory period becomes the limit. This is the principle of supramaximal stimulation valid for nerve membrane stimulation and MEPs (see below).

Stimulating Electrodes

The most commonly used stimulation side in the upper extremities is the median nerve, and for the lower extremities it is the tibial nerve. Details of placement are provided below. Important: place the anode 2 to 3 cm distal to the cathode to avoid an anodal block.

Detecting the SSEP Signal

The cortical signal is detected by electrodes which are placed according to the EEG system: the 10–20 system (▶ Fig. 7.1). Similar to the EEG setting, the scalp electrodes can be referred to a similar electrode (theoretically inactive) for all electrodes (referential montage) or to another active electrode (bipolar montage).

The bipolar electrodes are close together: they therefore record near-field responses and subtract far-field responses. They are best for analyzing low-to-medium amplitude waveforms that are localized. The referential montage, on the other hand, has the electrodes spaced far apart. Therefore, far-field responses are included. If the recording electrode is near the source generator in the referential system, the second electrode is usually far away and indifferent; therefore, a high-amplitude potential will be obtained. On the other hand, increasing electrode distance will also increase noise, most of all muscle artifacts.

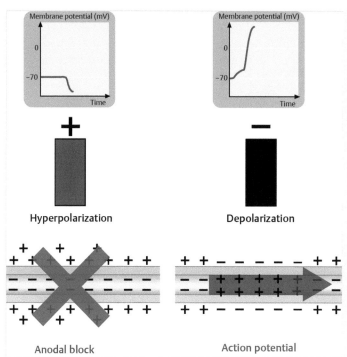

Fig. 7.8 Anodal block due to bipolar stimulation.

As already stated, the source of SSEPs is the synaptic activity of sensory neurons (i.e., thalamus, somatosensory cortex) and the action potential along axons (i.e., brachial plexus). SSEP, therefore, monitors stationary sources and traveling sources.

In a traveling source (AP running along a nerve), the recording electrodes will pick up the signal at different time points (the point when the signal passes the recording electrode), so the latency of the signal will change. This is called a traveling potential (amplitude same, latency different).

Stationary potentials are potentials that arise from fixed anatomical structures (i.e., synapses). They are generated at the same time and recorded at the same time, but at different distances: therefore, different amplitudes.

Nomenclature of SSEP "Waves": The waves are named N for negative and P for positive. A negative wave is called a peak, and a positive wave is called a valley. The number represents the latency. The amplitude is from peak to trough. For example, N20 is a negative wave (forming a peak) which occurs 20 ms after stimulation. P14 and P22 is a positive wave (forming a valley) which is detected 22 ms after stimulation. These findings would be typical for

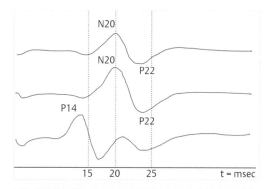

Fig. 7.9 Median nerve somatosensory-evoked potential (SSEP).

median nerve SSEPs (▶ Fig. 7.9). For tibial nerve SSEPs the signal will arrive later: P37 and N45 (▶ Fig. 7.10). Please note that these are idealized values: even in the healthy person latencies might be different. This will be compensated for by bilateral comparison and the principle of baseline recording. Important is to understand the dynamic changes during surgery. A typical "real life scenario" is demonstrated in ▶ **Video 7.1.**

7.3.3 How SSEPs Work—Details

We focus here on SSEP monitoring for supratentorial lesions.

Nerve stimulation is performed with constant-current stimulator.

SSEP monitoring is fairly standardized. We recommend to read in more depth.[2] Here is however a summary of the relevant details.

Placement of Stimulating Electrodes (▶ Video 7.2)

Tibial nerve: The cathode is positioned on the medial surface of the ankle, 1 to 2 cm distal and posterior to the medial malleolus. The anode should be placed 2 to 3 cm distal to the cathode (▶ Fig. 7.11).

Median nerve: The cathode is positioned between the tendons of the palmaris longus and the flexor carpi radialis muscles, 2 cm proximal to the wrist crease. The anode should be placed 2 to 3 cm distal to the cathode.

For safety reasons a grounding electrode should be placed, i.e., on the palmar surface of the forearm.

Stimulus Parameters

The nerves are stimulated with a monophasic rectangular pulse of 100 to 300 µs duration and 30 to 40 mA intensity.

Stimulus: A common repetition rate is around of 2–8/s. Stimulus rates must be optimized to obtain reliable responses in the shortest time possible. Fine adjustments of stimulus frequency are often necessary to eliminate noise artifacts.

System bandpass: System bandpass of 30 to 1 kHz is commonly used. Filter settings should be kept constant during a monitored procedure. Changes in filter settings will cause changes in the responses that can erroneously be attributed to pharmacologic or surgical factors. If filter settings are changed, it is important that baselines be reestablished.

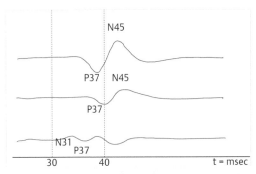

Fig. 7.10 Tibial nerve somatosensory-evoked potential (SSEP).

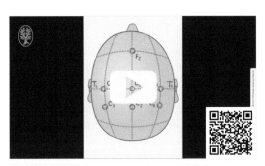

Video 7.2 Setup of SSEPS.

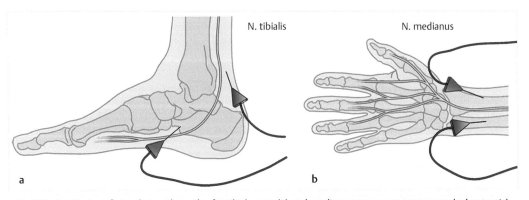

Fig. 7.11 Positioning of stimulating electrodes for tibial nerve (a) and median nerve somatosensory-evoked potential (SSEP) (b).

Analysis time: The analysis time should be at least twice the usual latency of the waveform of interest. Thus, in a median nerve SSEP, the last waveform of interest is the N20; therefore, the analysis for an upper limb study should be at least 40 to 50 ms.

Number of trials to be averaged: Approximately, 250 to 1000 repetitions are needed; the number of repetitions must be balanced between the quality of the signal and a potential delayed feedback to the surgeon.

Electrode type and placement: In the OR usually cork screw electrodes are used as they provide sufficient fixation and prevent dislocation due to draping and positional changes. For direct cortical recording a grid electrode can be placed on the cortical surface. Though this positioning can compensate for brain shift, the grid is notoriously susceptible to incidental displacements and changes of impedance due to irrigation and blood accumulation.

Montage: A minimum of four-channel recording is recommended. The nomenclature follows the 10–20 system; however, the SSEP electrodes are placed 2 centimeters behind (dorsal) and are designed with an additional bar: C3 becomes C3′, C4 becomes C4′... A contralateral (i.e., on the side of the stimulated nerve) scalp or ear electrode may serve as a reference.

▶ Fig. 7.12 reviews the placement of electrodes for a typical SSEP montage as used for cranial surgery. A cervical electrode (Cv1) is placed below the inion (▶ Fig. 7.13).

Analysis of results and criteria for cortical localization: Typically, N20/P30 waveforms are recorded over the somatosensory cortex whereas waveforms of the opposite polarity, P20/N30, are recorded over the primary motor cortex. Adjacent electrodes over the pre- and postcentral gyri demonstrate, thus, a "phase reversal" between the N20 and the P20. The localization of the phase reversal indicates the site of the central sulcus.

Warning criteria: SSEPs are characterized by amplitude and latency.[2] Alterations of SSEPs are reported immediately to the surgical team. Benign factors like displacement of the grid, change in position of the cortex in relation to the scalp electrodes or changes in anesthesiologic parameter must be ruled out immediately. Typically, a 50% drop in amplitude and a 10% prolongation in latency are considered a significant change in SSEPs.[3]

7.3.4 Performed Practice

First of all, morphology and latency of the waves depend on multiple factors, which will change during the operation. This is very different from SSEP test in the office with very stable conditions. It is, therefore, of utmost importance to get baseline before the intervention has started. Even with baselines the "textbook" expected, i.e., P37 or N45 (▶ Fig. 7.10) can be detected earlier or later without a pathological correlate (▶ Video 7.1, ▶ Fig. 7.14 and ▶ Fig. 7.15). It is also very important to have a side comparison as the not involved system serves as a control. It is also relevant to observe the SSEP

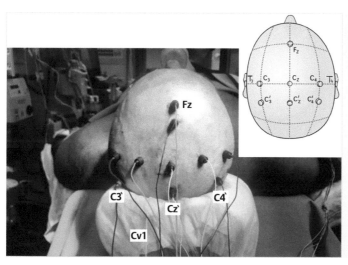

Fig. 7.12 Placement of electrodes for a typical somatosensory-evoked potential (SSEP) montage as used for cranial surgery: C3′, Cz′, C4′.

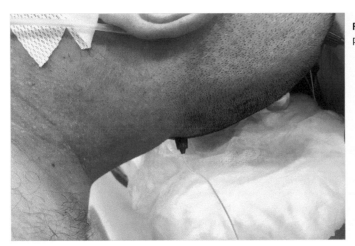

Fig. 7.13 A cervical electrode (Cv1) is placed below the inion.

signal from different "angles": Cz/Fz might give you a better amplitude than Cz/C4'.

Intraoperative Medianus SSEPs (▶ Fig. 7.14)—In this position C3'/4'-Fz will record the signal:
- N1 (N20) at around 20 ms.
- P1 (P25) at around 25 ms.

If a cervical electrode is used (Cv1) in reference to Fz, then N1 signal will be detected at around 12 ms.

Intraoperative tibialis SSEPs (▶ **Video 7.1** and ▶ Fig. 7.15):

Typical recording is by electrodes positioned in the midline (remember localization of the leg area) by electrode Cz' (2 cm behind Cz) referred to Fz.

In this position Cz'-Fz will record the signal:
- N33 at around 35 ms.
- P40 at around 41 ms.

If a cervical electrode is used (Cv1) in reference to Fz, then N1 signal will be detected at around 31 ms.

7.4 MEP

In a nutshell, motor-evoked potentials (MEPs) are recorded from muscles following transcranial or direct stimulation of motor cortex. An initial D (i.e., direct) wave is followed by several I (i.e., indirect) waves, which come at periodic intervals (usually about 1 ms). D waves represent the direct excitation of corticospinal tract neurons, while I waves reflect indirect depolarization of the same axons via corticocortical connections.

As these multiple volleys descend the corticospinal tracts, they summate at the anterior horn cells in the spinal cord. If the threshold is reached,

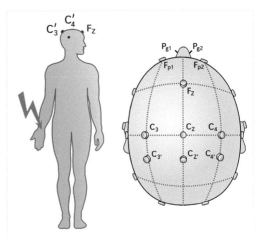

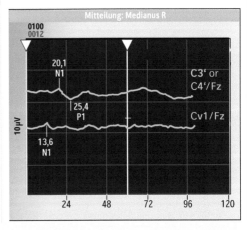

Fig. 7.14 Typical recording by electrodes positioned lateral (remember localization of the arm area) C3` or C4`Cz` (2 cm behind C3/4).

neuronal firing is induced and the corresponding muscle contracts. This CMAP is detected in the EMG and corresponds to a group of almost simultaneous action potentials from several muscle fibers in the same area.

7.4.1 How MEP Works—Principles

MEP works with either transcranial cortical or direct cortical and subcortical stimulation. We have already reviewed the principle of nerve stimulation; however, there are some differences performing CNS stimulation. The mechanism by which cortical/subcortical stimulation induces a measurable muscle contraction depends on a local induction of (in the end) action potentials.

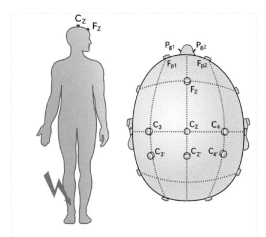

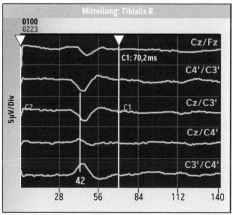

Fig. 7.15 Tibialis somatosensory-evoked potential (SSEP): note that the classical "N45" is seen at 42 ms. Note the different amplitudes for different angles (electrode position relative to the source).

Therefore, the neurostimulator needs to depolarize the membrane of pyramidal cells.

For cortical stimulation MEP works with anodal stimulation of the cortex. The cathode works as a reference (▶ Fig. 7.16). MEPs are always easiest to elicit and characterize when you use anodal, monopolar, pulse-train stimulation.[1]

One proposed mechanism is that anodal current enters (and hyperpolarizes) dendrites at the surface of the brain. We have reviewed the principles of this mechanism in the SSEP chapter as we discussed nerve stimulation (▶ Fig. 7.6 and ▶ Fig. 7.8). Simplified, anodal stimulation is just the injection of positively charged ions under the electrode (▶ Fig. 7.17). Because opposites attract, negatively charged ions migrate to the very surface of cortex under the anode. You can think of this as a **current sink** and the consequence is hyperpolarization of the apical dendrites of the pyramidal cell. In order to compensate for this current sink, a **current source** is generated distally such that positively charged ions congregate around the other end of the pyramidal cell. This results in depolarization (activation) of the cell body, the axon hillock, and the initial segment of the axon, which forms the corticospinal tract.

This works only if the "infusion" of cations "meets" the dendritical apex. So, there are three-dimensional considerations that you need to consider if you place your electrodes. For example, if you place the monopolar stimulating electrode over the motor cortex and deliver anodal stimulation to stimulate the hand area, your lowest

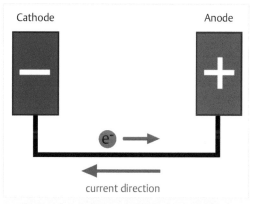

Fig. 7.16 For cortical stimulation motor-evoked potential (MEP) works with anodal stimulation of the cortex. The cathode works as a reference.

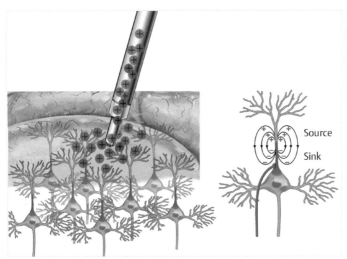

Fig. 7.17 The concept of cortical anodal stimulation; here with a monopolar stimulator as used for direct cortical stimulation. Injection of positively charged ions under the electrode induces hyperpolarization of the apical dendrites of the pyramidal cell.

Source

Sink

threshold CMAPs are from the vertically oriented cells just below your electrode at C3 or C4 (hand representation of the motor homunculus). To get MEPs from the legs by stimulating C3 or C4, an increase of intensity is necessary. This is because those "leg" cells are deep in the interhemispheric fissure and the cells are oriented horizontal to your anodal stimulating electrode.

7.4.2 How MEP Works—Details

Like with the SSEP monitoring, we recommend that you read in more depth. Here is, however, a summary of the relevant details.

Stimulation Equipment

The generator delivering the stimulation for transcranial electrical stimulation (TES) or direct cortical or subcortical stimulation should be able to deliver brief trains of high-intensity stimuli. It is important that the intensity of the stimulus pulses, the number of pulses per train, and the interpulse interval (or equivalently, the pulse rate) within the train can all be adjusted. Either constant-voltage or constant-current stimulators can be used. In constant-voltage stimulation, the stimulus current can vary widely depending on the impedance of the tissue and the electrode–tissue interface.

Transcranial Electrical Stimulation

Needle or corkscrew electrodes are most often used for TES. Corkscrew electrodes have low impe-

dances and are less likely to become dislodged. For the upper extremities, stimulating electrodes are placed at scalp positions C3/C4 of the 10–10 (expanded 10–20) system[4] (▶ Fig. 7.1 and ▶ Fig. 7.18, ▶ **Video 7.3**). For the lower extremities, electrodes at C3/C4 are used. The C3/C4 stimulating montages have the advantage that they can stimulate the motor pathways for both upper and lower limbs with a single stimulus train, permitting simultaneous recording of upper-limb and lower-limb MEPs. The Cz/Fz stimulating montage has the advantage that it may more reliably stimulate the motor pathways for the lower limbs bilaterally with a single stimulus. The optimal electrode arrangement for stimulation may vary between patients and surgical circumstances; different stimulation montages can be tested and the best one selected for each patient.

Recording Electrodes and Recording Sites

For the recording of D-waves you need to place paired electrodes near the spinal cord, either epidural or subdural. They may be placed percutaneously using a Touhy needle or placed by the surgeons within the surgical field. For the purpose of supratentorial resection, myogenic MEPs usually suffice and the invasive procedure necessary for recording of D-waves is not needed.

In the upper extremities, myogenic MEPs are optimally recorded from hand muscles (thenar, abductor digiti minimi, or first dorsal interosseous muscles) because of their being predominantly

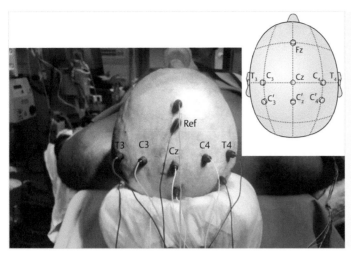

Fig. 7.18 Placement of electrodes for a typical motor-evoked potential (MEP) montage as used for cranial surgery: T3, C3, Cz, C4, T4, and reference electrode (Ref).

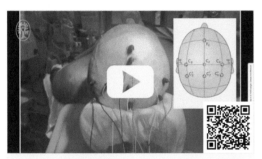

Video 7.3 Setup of MEPs.

under corticospinal tract control. More proximal muscles, i.e., biceps, can be used as well.

In the lower extremities, the tibialis anterior and abductor hallucis are the muscles most commonly used for myogenic MEP monitoring.

Measurements and Alarm Criteria

Alarm criteria based on latency are in general not useful during MEP monitoring.[5] Amplitude measurements are more useful in evaluating myogenic MEPs.

The amplitude of the myogenic MEP is measured between the most positive and the most negative points of the response waveform. Muscle MEP warning criteria are tailored to the type of surgery and based on deterioration clearly exceeding variability with no confounding factor explanation. Disappearance is always a major criterion. Major criteria for supratentorial monitoring include > 50%

amplitude reduction when warranted by sufficient preceding response stability.[6]

7.5 Electromyography (EMG)

In a nutshell, **electromyography** (**EMG**) is a technique for evaluating and recording the electrical activity produced by skeletal muscles. To perform EMG you need an **electromyograph** to produce an **electromyogram**. An electromyograph detects the electrical potential generated by muscle cells when these cells are activated (▶ Fig. 6.13). The signals can be analyzed to detect activation levels.

7.5.1 How EMG Works—Principles

Muscle activity is detected by electrodes placed on the surface near or (with a needle) into the target muscle. Normal muscles exhibit a brief burst of muscle fiber activation when stimulated by needle movement, but this rarely lasts more than 100 ms.

7.5.2 How EMG Works—Details

Apart from the stimulation-induced activity of the muscle, intraoperative applications of EMG are the continuous free-running EMG (very important in surgery putting brain nerves at risk) or the "triggered" EMG in which recording of the respective muscles is associated with the respective stimulus, thus filtered against spontaneous occurring signals.

As in routine EMG, an active and reference electrode must be placed in each channel. A single large lead ground can be used for all channels. Depending on the surgical procedure and the number of channels available, the recording and reference electrodes can be placed into the individual muscle of interest.

Recording Parameters

Usually, CMAPs are recorded with needle electrodes from target muscles in the face and the upper and lower extremities. Most commonly used muscles are orbicularis oris, mentalis, biceps, extensor, flexor, hypothenar, ID1, tibialis anterior, Abd hallucis. The signals are amplified 10,000 times and are recorded on epochs of 100 ms with a filter setting. CMAPs are amplified 10,000 times and are recorded during a 100 ms epoch with a 1.5 to 853 Hz filter setting. Baseline recordings are obtained after positioning of the patient on the operating table.

References

[1] Vogel R. Understanding anodal and cathodal stimulation. 2017 https://www.asnm.org/blogpost/1635804/290597/Understanding-Anodal-and-Cathodal-Stimulation. Accessed July 12, 2020

[2] American Clinical Neurophysiological Society. Guideline 11B: recommended standards for intraoperative monitoring of somatosensory evoked potentials. 2006https://www.acns.org/pdf/guidelines/Guideline-11B.pdf. Accessed July 12, 2020

[3] Nuwer MR, Packwood JW. Somatosensory evoked potential monitoring with scalp and cervical recording. In: Nuwer MR, ed. Handbook of Clinical Neurophysiology 8, Elsevier; 2008

[4] American Electroencephalographic Society. American Electroencephalographic Society guidelines in electroencephalography, evoked potentials, and polysomnography. J Clin Neurophysiol. 1994; 11(1):1–147

[5] Deletis V, Sala F. Intraoperative neurophysiological monitoring of the spinal cord during spinal cord and spine surgery: a review focus on the corticospinal tracts. Clin Neurophysiol. 2008; 119(2):248–264

[6] Macdonald DB, Skinner S, Shils J, Yingling C, American Society of Neurophysiological Monitoring. Intraoperative motor evoked potential monitoring: a position statement by the American Society of Neurophysiological Monitoring. Clin Neurophysiol. 2013; 124(12):2291–2316

8 Direct Cortical and Subcortical Mapping

8.1 The Scope of This Chapter

After having laid out the principles of IONM, we are now considering the direct, invasive aspects of IONM, which is the most relevant part of this book for neurosurgeons. It is quite evident that the introduction of technology that gives the neurosurgeon the option to directly evaluate the functionality of the tissue (that he is about to destroy…) was a game changer. This is dramatically important for the concept of supramarginal resection, where infiltrated but potentially functional tissue becomes the target of resection. **The fundamental principle of this technique is the identification of functionality and,** maybe even more important **the exclusion of functionality**. As we have now clear evidence for the impact of resection, IONM not only becomes a modus that is used to prevent the surgeon from inducing deficits, but becomes a strong ally to push the resection to the functional limit. In this cutting-edge situation, in which the neurosurgeon needs to consider whether to resect or not, interpretation of IONM findings often tip the scale. It is therefore obvious that a profound understanding of the technique of direct cortical and subcortical stimulation is indispensable for neurooncological neurosurgery.

8.2 Direct Cortical and Subcortical Mapping: Principles

One of the principal problems when interfering with the electricity of the brain is that the cortex and the surrounding structures have irregular geometries and inhomogeneous electrical properties. Add the fact of the additional pathology (tumor tissue of variant density and edema), the distribution of electric field and current density generated during cortical and subcortical stimulation, the actual functionality of the tissue cannot be easily predicted. It is also unclear how the distribution of the electric field and current affect the different neuronal elements in the cortex, because cortical neurons vary in shape, size, location, and orientation. Electrode polarity, electrode position, and stimulation parameter have a large and distinct influence on the response of cortical and subcortical neural elements to stimuli.

Nevertheless, cortical and subcortical stimulation work (somehow), but as we will see, they are not always a precise and exactly reproducible method.

There are two options for surgical cortical and subcortical stimulation: **low-frequency** (bipolar) and **high-frequency** (monopolar) stimulation. Both methods are based on one endpoint: to avoid false-negative stimulation (as you would be unaware that you are removing eloquent structures…). Therefore, the principle of positive control is crucial. Positive control provides confidence that a negative stimulation is a true negative: hence the tissue is resectable without inducing a deficit. As the parameters that influence electrophysiological parameter (depth of anesthesia, alertness, etc.) might change in due course. Therefore, the exposure of cortical areas in which positive control is obtainable is (probably) mandatory. The most reliable way to obtain a positive control is to expose the M1 (motor) cortex, as stimulation-induced response is most reliably induced in these areas[1,2,3,4,5,6] (▶ Fig. 8.1). This means, that even if the lesion is not located in the vicinity of M1 (i.e., located in the frontal area), you need to consider to extend the craniotomy far behind the coronal suture.

8.3 High-frequency Stimulation/Monopolar Stimulation: Principles

High-frequency stimulation[7] uses a monopolar probe with a reference electrode, which is usually located at the FZ position. Therefore, the brain is exposed to a large electrical field that extends

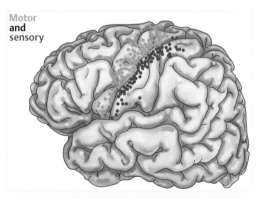

Fig. 8.1 Motor functions (*green*) can serve as a positive control on both hemispheres. Data correspond to intraoperative stimulation points accumulated during the past decades by several authors.

from the stimulation site to the reference electrode, exposing not only the cortical contact site but also the subcortical structures to an electrical field (▶ Fig. 8.2 and ▶ Fig. 8.3). Either the tip of the stimulator or the reference electrode might serve as anode or cathode. Monopolar stimulation is therefore optional as anodal-cathodal or cathodal-anodal stimulation.

Important point: It is important to note that cathodal-anodal and anodal-cathodal stimulations have different effects on the stimulated tissue.

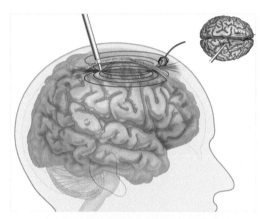

Fig. 8.2 By monopolar stimulation, the brain is exposed to a large electrical field that extends from the stimulation site to the reference electrode.

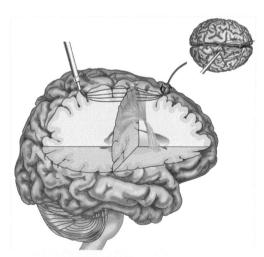

Fig. 8.3 Monopolar stimulation exposes not only the cortical contact site but also the subcortical structures to an electrical field.

The response evoked by high frequency is an MEP resulting in a CMAP of the respective muscles. Therefore, monopolar stimulation is associated with the use of an electromyography machine.

Anodal-cathodal cortical stimulation triggers a **cortical** motor response with lower stimulation intensity as compared to cathodal-anodal stimulation or bipolar stimulation.[8] As first demonstrated by Ranck, a motor response by stimulation of myelinated fiber (i.e., cortical spinal tract) took less cathodal than anodal current.[8] In a clinical study, Cedzich reported that monophasic anodal stimulus was better for cortical stimulation than for brain stem stimulation. Conversely, a monophasic cathodal stimulus was more effective for brain stem stimulation.[9]

In simple words:

Clinical application: Anodal-cathodal stimulation is used for eliciting cortical motor response. Cathodal-anodal stimulation is used for eliciting subcortical motor responses.

8.4 Low-Frequency/Bipolar Stimulation: Principles

In contrast to high-frequency stimulation, in bipolar stimulation cathode and anode are at a much smaller distance separated by 5 to 10 mm. The charge density applied to the brain is located between the tips. This induces an almost homogenous and localized electrical field (▶ Fig. 8.4). Therefore, the bipolar technique provides a higher

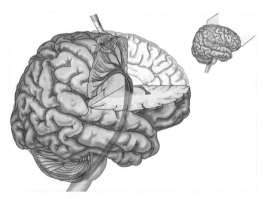

Fig. 8.4 In bipolar stimulation cathode and anode are at a much smaller distance separated by 5 to 10 mm. The charge density applied to the brain is located between the tips. This induces an almost homogenous and localized electrical field.

resolution map of the surface being stimulated as compared to monopolar stimulation. Though it is possible to trigger an MEP with bipolar stimulation, the stimulation intensity needed to trigger an MEP is very high (up to 40 mA as compared to <12 mA for high-frequency stimulation), thus putting the patient at high risk for seizures. At lower intensity, bipolar stimulation blocks neuronal functions. Therefore, this is the method of choice for sensory and language mapping in the awake setting.

The neurophysiological background of the block of neurological functions by bipolar stimulation (▶ Fig. 8.5) is not well understood. One possible explanation is the induction of an anodal block.

Thus, when bipolar electrodes are placed in the same orientation as a fiber, a fiber will be depolarized under the cathode, and hyperpolarized under the anode. If the hyperpolarization is large enough, an action potential initiated under the cathode may not be able to propagate through the region of hyperpolarization. If this is the case, the action

potential will propagate in only one direction. If this direction is not heading toward the descending axon this might result in a block of the signal transduction, thus inducing a block of functions, similar to an anodal block as observed in peripheral nerve stimulation (▶ Fig. 7.8).

Both methods are highly susceptible to factors that might change during surgery like temperature, depth of anesthesia, awareness state of the patients, blood pressure, etc. As these factors cannot always be controlled, it is, as already said, advisable to have a positive control, which defines the threshold for the stimulation parameter needed in the individual patient in the individual time.

Clinical application: In simple words: you need to define the parameter which gives you a block of function (low-frequency stimulation—bipolar stimulation) or a stimulation of muscle activity (high-frequency stimulation—monopolar stimulation) before you decide that the tissue is resectable due to your stimulation findings. Once you have defined a positive stimulation point, you need to define the threshold: the lowest stimulation intensity, which still gives you a clear response. Again to this end it is very useful to expose, i.e., the M1 motor cortex, define your parameters there, and then go back to your resection site. This is the principle of positive mapping.

8.5 Direct Cortical and Subcortical Mapping: Details

Both methods are associated with an increased rate of intraoperative seizures (LF >> HF). Though these can be blocked by administration of barbiturates, this is for obvious reasons undesirable. The most efficient way to stop a seizure is ice-cold saline. Make sure that you have at least 5 L of ice-cold saline or Ringer's solution for irrigation to abrogate an induced seizure during stimulation.

8.6 High-Frequency Stimulation: Details

High-frequency stimulation is performed with a monopolar probe toward a reference electrode, usually in the asleep setting. The stimulus has a monophasic form, a duration of 0.5 ms, and it can be administered as a train of stimuli (generally 5: train of 5) separated by 3 ms (the interstimulus interval),

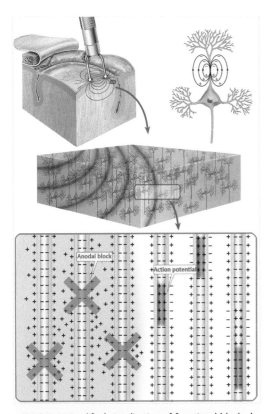

Fig. 8.5 A simplified visualization of functional blocked cortical areas by bipolar stimulation.

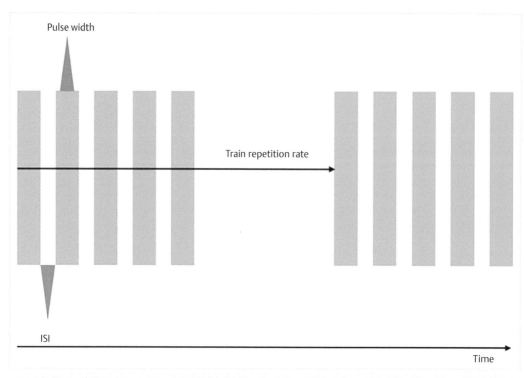

Fig. 8.6 "Train of 5" technique: 3 ms (=250 Hz) inter-stimulus interval (ISI), pulse width 0.5 ms, 5 pulses within a train.

and delivered every 1 s (repetition rate: 1 Hz) or every 2 s (repetition rate: 0.5 Hz) (▶ Fig. 8.6).

Responses induced by monopolar stimulation are MEPs; therefore, this method is limited to the monitoring of the motor system. Responses are evaluated with an electromyograph. MEP monitoring (in contrast to bipolar stimulation) provides both qualitative (type or group of muscle evoked) and quantitative parameters (MEP amplitude, latency, and current intensity). As already mentioned, a fundamental concept during stimulation is the identification of the stimulation threshold. This means that the lowest current intensity, evoking a detectable motor response, is defined. This stimulation threshold must be identified both at the cortical and the subcortical levels and necessitates the surgical exposure of this area, even if this area is not involved in the planned resection. Usually, hand muscle MEPs are identified at 3 to 7 mA in the awake patient and around 9 to 12 mA in the asleep patient. In the subcortical setting, high frequency allows for an approximation of the distance from the motor fibers. In the case of the use of high frequency, there is a relationship between the amount of current delivered by the stimulator and the distance from the motor tract (1 mA of current used for stimulation and 1 mm of distance from the corticospinal tract; 1 mA–1 mm rule, see paper[10]).

Important point: As the impedance within the resection cavity might dynamically change (blood, air, irrigation), you need to be very cautious with this rule.

However, a subcortical stimulation threshold of 3 to 5 mA is the minimum recommended to achieve a safe resection and not to endanger the motor tract.

Clinical application: Consider stopping the resection if you get a subcortical, positive response with 3 to 5 mA. However, this is highly dependent on the individual situation, especially the determined threshold on the cortical site and the individual oncological situation: are you resecting a high-grade gliomas or is it a low-grade glioma? Would the patient accept a surgically induced deficit for a better resection?

8.7 High-Frequency Monitoring with a Grid Electrode

Apart from the intermittent testing with the monopolar probe, the placing of a grid electrode on the primary motor areas enables a continuous MEPs. Stimulation parameters are the same as described for standard monopolar motor mapping.

The advantage of the grid is the direct placement on the cortical surface, therefore avoiding the technical problems of transcranial MEP. Intraoperative, transcranial MEPs suffer from varying distance of the scalp electrodes toward the motor cortex due to the displacement of the relevant structures in the respective phases of surgery. This system is an effective way to monitoring the activity of motor pathways (from the cortex to the effector) and it is sensitive for any vascular damage. This method is particularly useful during resection of deep-seated lesion with a close relationship with vascular structures (i.e., insular gliomas and anterior perforating arteries).

Any changes of MEPs are reported by the neurophysiologist to the surgeon, who can initiate maneuvers (such as irrigation of the vessels and increasing the mean arterial pressure) trying to obtain a recovery of the MEPs and thus avoiding vascular damage.

8.8 Low-Frequency Stimulation—Details

Awake surgery begins with the determination of tasks that need to be tested according to the specific localization of the lesion. The patient is then informed about the details of the procedure. It is mandatory that the patient is well informed and motivated. The chosen tasks are trained, preferably in a simulated setting.

Low-frequency stimulation (aka bipolar stimulation, 50 or 60 Hz) is almost exclusively associated with awake craniotomy. Different regiments can be used: complete awake, asleep–awake, and asleep–awake–asleep. A field block with, (i.e., bupivacaine) 0.5% with epinephrine 0.0005% is placed near the sensory nerves of the scalp (▶ Fig. 8.7). Insertion points of the head clamp must be blocked as well (▶ Fig. 8.8). The planned incision is infiltrated as well.

The settings of the bipolar stimulator are summarized in ▶ Fig. 8.9.

In asleep–awake and asleep–awake–asleep cases, a laryngeal mask is used to ensure patient ventilation. Generally, before the incision is made midazolam (2 mg; avoided if an electroencephalogram is to be recorded) and fentanyl (50–100 mg) are administered. During surgery, either

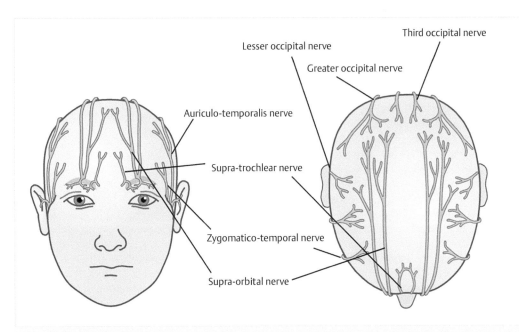

Fig. 8.7 Localization of sensory nerves of the head. Field blocks should be administered as small depots in their vicinity.

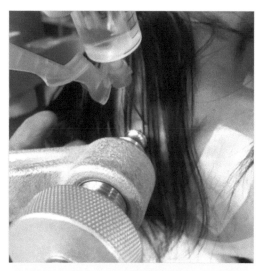

Fig. 8.8 Insertion points of the head clamp should be blocked as well.

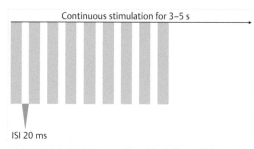

Fig. 8.9 Bipolar stimulation parameters (low-frequency stim): biphasic pulse of <1 ms or 1 to 4 s pulse series.

propofol (50–100 mg/kg of body weight per minute; avoided if an electroencephalogram is to be recorded) or dexmedetomidine (0.2–0.7 mg/kg/h) and remifentanil (0.05–0.2 mg/kg/min) are given. Once the craniotomy is performed, the dura can be anesthetized along either side of the middle meningeal artery. Anesthetic agents are stopped as soon as the surgeon has established the approach to the tumor, and the high intracranial pressure (palpation of the dura) is excluded and the dura opened.

As soon as the patient is sufficiently cooperative, motor mapping is performed to establish the threshold. Initial parameters include 1 to 2 mA, with a frequency of 60 Hz and a pulse duration of 1 ms. Stimulus intensity should be increased in 0.5-mA steps. Amplitudes of greater than 4 mA are not recommended in motor cortex stimulation. Stimulating different areas in sequence rather than immediately adjacent areas and using pauses of at least 10 seconds between stimulations decreases the risk of intraoperative seizures.

Cortical patches of 1 cm³ are stimulated sequentially with rest periods between stimulations (▶ Fig. 8.10). The probe is applied to the cortex for 3 to 5 seconds and changes in the motor performances are noted. As soon as the motor threshold is established, language testing or sensory mapping can be performed. Language mapping is done in the awake patient when the lesion involves the dominant perisylvian frontotemporal region or the subcortical white matter tracts. Intraoperative language mapping is not useful in patients with significant language deficits. Cortical patches of 5 mm are stimulated sequentially with rest periods between stimulations. The probe is applied to the cortex for 1 to 3 seconds and the patient is monitored. Each cortical patch is tested up to three times. For each site, the patient is tested for counting errors, object naming errors, and word reading errors as they are presented on naming cards. A cortical area is considered positive for language function if the patient is unable to count, name objects, repeat words, or read words in two out of three stimulations. Speech arrest can be attributed to a stimulus disturbance of language function or arrest of motor activity. After exposure of subcortical structures subcortical stimulation mapping is performed, using stimulation parameters that are generally similar to cortical mapping but higher amplitudes can be needed. Once thresholds for motor activation are identified, repeated stimulations in this area are performed to confirm that motor threshold has not changed. Thus, obtaining a baseline threshold of activation as reference is very important.

8.9 Focus: How to Test Language Intraoperatively

For basic intraoperative testing of language[11] and visual mapping[12,13] we suggest:
- Speech planning and articulation (i.e., speech arrest and verbal apraxia):
  - Counting test (or series repetition) for assessing of[14,15,16] anomia, semantic, or phonological paraphasia.
  - Object naming for language (i.e., adapted national version of Boston DO80[14,17,18] for words and nonwords) or phrases reading.[19]

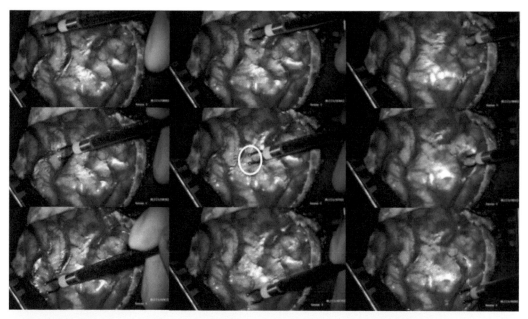

Fig. 8.10 Cortical patches of 1 cm³ are stimulated sequentially with rest periods between stimulations.

- Visual system:
  - Object naming in quadrants separated by dotted line for positive (phosphenes, color flashes, etc.) and negative.
- Semantic association:
  - Test pyramid and palm tree test (PPTT) for monitoring of nonverbal comprehension in the hemisphere that is nonspecialized in language. For a sample, see also ▶ Table 8.1.

A crucial step in language testing is the differentiation between anomia (trouble in semantic retrieval) and anarthria (speech output block). This is possible by asking the patient to introduce the object naming by using a carrier sentence: i.e., "this is" before the object naming. This is of special importance at the level of the crucial cortical epicenters for SAN (in particular, VPMC in the frontal lobe and SMG and AG in the parietal lobe) or in the white matter of the ventral frontoparietal junction (i.e., corresponding to the course of SLF III). Finally, it is crucial to distinguish between a real speech arrest (i.e., anarthria) and a trouble in speech output due to the stimulation of the orofacial motor area. Speech arrest is, in fact, a block in language production with preserved ability to move orofacial muscle. It is often induced by stimulation of the cortex just anterior to the face motor area.

8.9.1 Temporo-Parieto-Occipital Junction

The stimulation of the temporo-parieto-occipital junction should be routinely used to assess the position of the following bundles and terminations: SLF III, vertical SLF, and deeply the AF (in particular, its descending vertical position). For these reasons, the most frequent functional responses at the cortical levels are: Speech arrest or verbal apraxia due to the stimulation of termination of SLF III (or cortical hubs of the SAN)[16] particularly at the level of the SMG and AG (▶ Fig. 8.11); anomia or semantic disturbances due to deactivation of the phonologico-sematic integration at the temporo-parietal junction, or to sensory integration (subserved by the transversal fiber of vertical SLF and VOF) (▶ Fig. 8.12); phonological paraphasia due to the stimulation of the terminations of AF or of cortical epicenters of this subnetwork largely distributed also within the temporal lobe (▶ Fig. 8.13).

At subcortical level the same functional responses should be expected and these functions tested in order to define the course of the SLF III in the dorsal part (i.e., parietal resection), AF, and vertical SLF and VOF fibers in the more temporal-centered resection. Finally, it is crucial to define the deep limit of resection to identify in both regions (dorsal and ventral)

Table 8.1 A sample of different and basic tasks for testing language during awake surgery

Counting test	counting 0 ... 10
Object naming	this is
Naming in quadrants	this is + this is
Words and non-words reading	**BOOK**
Pyramid and palm tree test	

the fibers of the IFOF evoking semantic paraphasia and anomia at DES, which constitute the deep functional limit of this resection (▶ Fig. 8.14).

8.9.2 Temporo-Occipital, Temporo-Basal, and Occipital Resections

For more ventral resections (i.e., temporo-occipital junction) or access to temporo-basal lesions, a full language cortical mapping, as previously described, is mandatory in addition to a reading test. Testing for alexia is crucial considering both the cortical territories of termination of ILF, the location of the VWFA, and, deeply, to reach more deeper seated lesion without damaging the ILF fibers (▶ Fig. 8.15).

Even in case of temporo-basal and deep-seated lesion, testing language (with object naming) is crucial to identify the superior limit of resection,

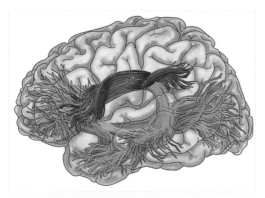

Fig. 8.11 Schematic representation of the course of SLF III fibers in the lateral white matter connecting the frontal parietal opercula. The stimulation in this region produces systematic verbal apraxia (i.e., articulatory disorders) during language production (i.e., counting or repeating series) (SLF, superior longitudinal fascicle).

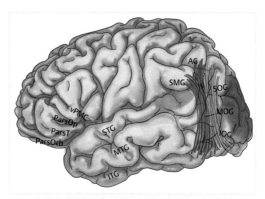

Fig. 8.12 Schematic representation of the transverse fibers of the temporo-parietal junction (i.e., vertical SLF and VOF, purple and green, respectively). The stimulation in this area induces frequently anomia. (SLF, superior longitudinal fascicle; VOF, vertical occipital fascicle).

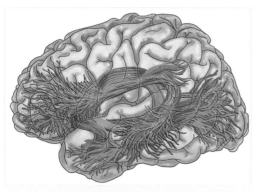

Fig. 8.13 Schematic representation of the AF course. The stimulation of this perisylvian white matter induces frequently phonological paraphasia (AF, arcuate fascicle).

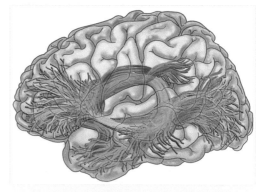

Fig. 8.14 In this figure the ventral course of IFOF fibers from the occipital and parietal lobe to the frontal lobe is highlighted. The stimulation of this long-range fiber all over their course produces systematically semantic paraphasia or anomia, due to deactivation of the semantic network (IFOF, inferior fronto-occipital fascicle).

i.e., the fibers of IFOF (eliciting semantic paraphasia and/or anomia when in contact with DES) (▶ Fig. 8.16).

Even if pure resections of the occipital lobe, and in particular involving the calcarine cortices, are rare, cortical DES in this area (eliciting visual responses, i.e., phosphenes) can be very useful to map the anterosuperior and mediolateral extension of the resection with respect to the expected visual field sacrifice. Reducing the visual field deficit to a quadrantopsia should be considered in order to reduce the impact of this deficit on the quality of life of patients (e.g., drive license, work activities, etc.).[12,13]

8.9.3 Visual and Acoustic Pathways Mapping

The stimulation of projection pathways particularly of OR all over its course induces phosphenes; the topographical distribution of phosphenes by dotted cross line (see possible testing in ▶ Table 8.2) provides useful information about whether the region of the OR (superior or inferior) is stimulated and thus it is particularly useful for sculpturing the resection avoiding hemianopia deficit.[12] The stimulation of AR is more difficult and no evidences of

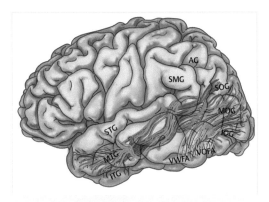

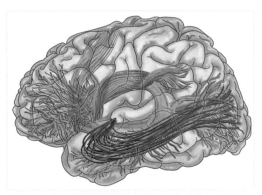

Fig. 8.15 In this figure we resumed the full course of ILF. The stimulation of the posterior portion of these fibers (in *yellow*) induces reading troubles (i.e., alexia) (ILF, inferior longitudinal fascicle).

Fig. 8.16 In this figure the course of the optic radiation (*red*) is highlighted in respect to the association pathways of the dorsal and the ventral stream. In particular, the superior portion of the optic radiation is covered by the fibers of the IFOF (IFOF, inferior fronto-occipital fascicle).

Table 8.2 Two possible tests for monitoring the visual field: the picture naming in opposite quadrants, and a white screen with dotted line separating the four quadrants of the visual field; both allow to monitor the distribution of the phosphenes between the superior and inferior quadrants during stimulation

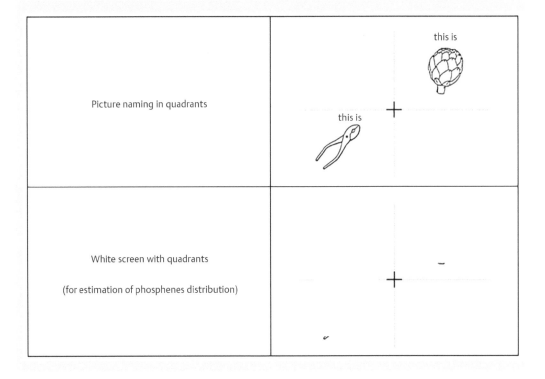

major neurological impairment due to resection of AR on one hemisphere are reported. However, the stimulation on the temporal side of the most superior and posterior portion of the temporo-opercular region (in correspondence of the HG) can elicit acoustic responses.[20]

References

[1] Berger MS, Ojemann GA. Intraoperative brain mapping techniques in neuro-oncology. Stereotact Funct Neurosurg. 1992; 58(1–4):153–161

[2] Berger MS. Functional mapping-guided resection of low-grade gliomas. Clin Neurosurg. 1995; 42:437–452

[3] Rasmussen T, Penfield W. Further studies of the sensory and motor cerebral cortex of man. Fed Proc. 1947; 6(2): 452–460

[4] Penfield W, Welch K. Instability of motor points and sensory points in the human cerebral cortex. Fed Proc. 1948; 7(1 Pt):91

[5] Fulton J. A note on the definition of the "motor" and "premotor" areas. Brain. 1935; 58(2):311–316

[6] Vogt C, Vogt O. Die vergleichend-architektonische und die vergleichend-reizphysiologische Felderung der Großhirnrinde unter besonderer Berücksichtigung der menschlichen. Naturwissenschaften. 1926; 14:1190–1194

[7] Kombos T, Süss O. Neurophysiological basis of direct cortical stimulation and applied neuroanatomy of the motor cortex: a review. Neurosurg Focus. 2009; 27(4):E3

[8] Ranck JB, Jr. Which elements are excited in electrical stimulation of mammalian central nervous system: a review. Brain Res. 1975; 98(3):417–440

[9] Cedzich C, Pechstein U, Schramm J, Schäfer S. Electrophysiological considerations regarding electrical stimulation of motor cortex and brain stem in humans. Neurosurgery. 1998; 42(3):527–532

[10] Nossek E, Korn A, Shahar T, et al. Intraoperative mapping and monitoring of the corticospinal tracts with neurophysiological assessment and 3-dimensional ultrasonography-based navigation. Clinical article. J Neurosurg. 2011; 114(3): 738–746

[11] Mandonnet E, Sarubbo S, Duffau H. Proposal of an optimized strategy for intraoperative testing of speech and language during awake mapping. Neurosurg Rev. 2017; 40 (1):29–35

[12] Sarubbo S, De Benedictis A, Milani P, et al. The course and the anatomo-functional relationships of the optic radiation: a combined study with "post mortem" dissections and 'in vivo' direct electrical mapping. J Anat. 2015; 226 (1):47–59

[13] Gras-Combe G, Moritz-Gasser S, Herbet G, Duffau H. Intraoperative subcortical electrical mapping of optic radiations in awake surgery for glioma involving visual pathways. J Neurosurg. 2012; 117(3):466–473

[14] Sarubbo S, Tate M, De Benedictis A, et al. Mapping critical cortical hubs and white matter pathways by direct electrical stimulation: an original functional atlas of the human brain. Neuroimage. 2020; 205:116237

[15] Tate MC, Herbet G, Moritz-Gasser S, Tate JE, Duffau H. Probabilistic map of critical functional regions of the human cerebral cortex: Broca's area revisited. Brain. 2014; 137 (Pt 10):2773–2782

[16] Zacà D, Corsini F, Rozzanigo U, et al. Whole-brain network connectivity underlying the human speech articulation as emerged integrating direct electric stimulation, resting state fMRI and tractography. Front Hum Neurosci. 2018; 12:405

[17] Duffau H, Gatignol P, Mandonnet E, Peruzzi P, Tzourio-Mazoyer N, Capelle L. New insights into the anatomo-functional connectivity of the semantic system: a study using cortico-subcortical electrostimulations. Brain. 2005; 128(Pt 4):797–810

[18] Sarubbo S, Tate M, De Benedictis A, et al. A normalized dataset of 1821 cortical and subcortical functional responses collected during direct electrical stimulation in patients undergoing awake brain surgery. Data Brief. 2019; 28: 104892

[19] Zemmoura I, Herbet G, Moritz-Gasser S, Duffau H. New insights into the neural network mediating reading processes provided by cortico-subcortical electrical mapping. Hum Brain Mapp. 2015; 36(6):2215–2230

[20] Roux FE, Lubrano V, Lauwers-Cances V, Trémoulet M, Mascott CR, Démonet JF. Intra-operative mapping of cortical areas involved in reading in mono- and bilingual patients. Brain. 2004; 127(Pt 8):1796–1810

9 Checklist for Awake Procedure

In the following, the essential practical details of an awake procedure (elective surgical indication) are presented in the form of a checklist.

Step 1: Evaluation of the patient
1. Suitability for awake operation:
   – Are there neurological deficits? (Is it possible to test the vulnerable functions?).
   – Is there a language barrier? (Is a translator needed?).
   – Is good compliance foreseeable? (Primary aggressive or depressive patient?).
2. Does the patient accept the perspective of an intraoperative awake phase?

Step 2: Preoperative Evaluation of Imaging
1. Where is the process related to potential functional cortical and subcortical areas?
   – Further imaging (fiber path imaging/nTMS) necessary?
   – Definition of endangered neurological functions (speech, motor skills).
   – Are these functions testable?
2. Definition of the operative goal in consensus with the patient and evaluation of acceptance of potential deficits in his current life situation. Preparing the patient for temporary deficits.

Step 3: Determine the surgical strategy
1. Which brain areas are tested for which functions?
2. Definition of the cortical and subcortical areas to be exposed and tested during resection.
3. Therefore define:
   – Necessary tests (language: image recognition, motor skills: line bisection test, Tapping board, fine motor exercises).
   – Position and size of the bone flap.
   – Skin incision.
   – Patient positioning.

Step 4: Preparing the Patient
1. Creating a relationship of trust with the patient through relaxed and open conversation.
2. Detailed explanation of the processes:
   – Schedule.
   – Bladder catheter.
   – Fixation of the head.
   – Sounds.
   – Positioning.

3. Simulation of intraoperative positioning.
4. Execution of planned tests in planned storage position.
   – Need glasses?
   – Hearing aid?
   – Tolerance of positioning in case of existing restrictions (Herniated disc, coxarthrosis).
5. Quantitative assessment of test results and re-evaluation of feasibility.

Step 5: Patient Positioning
1. Are all technical aids available?
   – Prepared table and position?
   – Devices such as navigation, ultrasound, ultrasound aspirator available and prepared?
   – Is local anesthesia available?
   – Is the microscope calibrated?
   – Is the stimulation device ready for use?
2. Has the local anesthesia been set up at the defined positions? Have Mayfield thorns and skin incision been infiltrated?
3. Conclusion of patient positioning only after consensus with the anesthesiologist: ventilation and option of reintubation checked and given?
4. Administration of mannitol necessary?
5. Sufficient amount of ice water in the room?

Step 6: Skin Incision and Craniotomy
1. Mental visualization of incision and planned craniotomy—Sufficient exposure?
2. Checking the cover:
   – Sufficient access to respiratory tract?
   – Tests possible (eyes free? Arms mobile?)?
3. Current surgical and anesthesia team informed about the process?
4. Procedure for epileptic seizures (ice-water rinsing) discussed?
5. After removal of the bone palpatory check intracranial pressure: if necessary countermeasures such as mannitol or modification of positioning.
6. Sufficient exposure? (Transdural use ultrasound/navigation).
7. Release of the waking phase by the surgeon.
8. Prepare a possible counteraction of a brain prolapse by tailoring a Tabotamb-piece as protection of the cortex with possibly necessary back pressure by the bone cover.

Step 7: Initial Waking Phase
1. Does it come to a brain prolapse by pressing or coughing?
2. Visualization of the planned access into the tumor by ultrasound/navigation.
3. Localization of the planned corticotomy.
4. Is the patient sufficiently cooperative and oriented to begin the testing?
5. Start stimulation only after tests have been successfully completed.
6. Silence in the operating room: communication channels between the surgeon, the patient, and the monitoring team have priority.

Step 8: Resection
1. Cortical mapping with definition of a positive control.
2. Retest the area of the planned corticotomy.

3. Is the patient still sufficiently compliant to do the test during the resection? Observe dynamics.
4. Start of stimulation and resection only with reproducible tests.
5. For resection cortical to subcortical mental visualization of the fiber tracts.
6. Selection of the tests to be performed according to the assumed anatomy.

Step 9: Complete the Resection
1. Perform final test.
2. Evaluation of the degree of alertness and the pain situation.
3. Consensus with anesthesia, whether slight sedation is sufficient or more anesthesia is necessary.
4. Transfer protocol with note that a progressive neurological disorder may occur.

Part C

The Practical Part

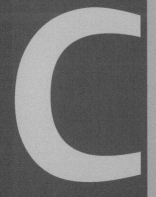

10 Introduction to the Practical Part

In Part B we have laid the groundwork for the practical application of IONM. In this practical part we will now put theory into practice. We will do this with a case-based approach. Based on the clinical history and preoperative imaging, we will systematically plan the procedure and define plan A and also a plan B. Though this book is focused on monitoring, we also need to discuss some aspects of resection techniques. We will present a video case which is only edited to avoid redundancy but demonstrates the real-life situation. To increase the didactic effect, we will ask you to assess the cases by yourself first, get your own plan, and then compare your approach to ours.

11 Finding the Indication for Surgery

11.1 Decision-Making in Neurooncological Neurosurgery

The decision-making process in surgery for infiltrating brain tumors has become very complicated, as we need to counterbalance the necessary aggressivity of resection with preservation of functionality (see also Chapter 4). The fundamental principle of your approach to the patient is a multiple-step process which is explained in ▶ Video 11.1.

11.2 A Systematical Approach to Evaluate the Indication for Surgery

11.2.1 Analyze the Lesion

In most cases a standard MRI with contrast series will be sufficient.

Go through these considerations:
- Is the lesion eloquent?
- What are the functions at risk?
- Localization of functions: cortical and subcortical (usually a combination).
- Are there vascular risks?

Identify the cortical and subcortical areas in which you will encounter "testable" areas. These have been well defined during the past decades. For your review, in ▶ Fig. 11.1a, b we have summarized

the established cortical stimulation points for the left and right hemisphere. In ▶ Fig. 11.2 we have summarized the subcortical "testable" areas.

11.2.2 Run Through Your IONM Options

- Which tests can be used to identify functions at risk?
- Are these tests in this patient feasible?

11.2.3 Risk Assessment

- What are the risks for a permanent deficit due to surgery?
- What is the natural course of the disease regarding the occurrence of deficits?

Are there alternative or adjuvant options to surgery?

Most of these assessments can be done based on the MRI scans. Please consider the MRI scans in ▶ Fig. 11.3. Let's assume the patient is 54 years, male, no neurological deficits, otherwise healthy. Define the eloquent anatomy (outline the cortical and subcortical areas of concern) and run through the list in Sections 11.2.1 and 11.2.2. As you integrate the three aspects (anatomy/testing functionality/risk assessment) you will have a plan. In ▶ Fig. 11.4 we have (crudely) sketched the potential functional areas of concern. In ▶ Fig. 11.5 we have added the

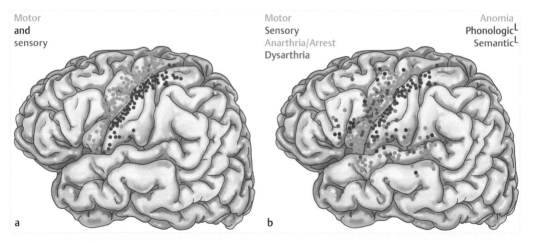

Fig. 11.1 Cortical areas corresponding to testable functions. **(a)** Left and right hemisphere. **(b)** Language dominant hemisphere (compare ▶ Fig. 8.1).

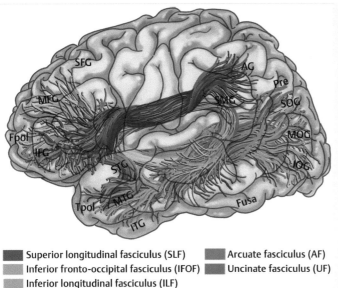

Fig. 11.2 Subcortical functional tracts. See Section 5.5 for correlation with language.

- ■ Superior longitudinal fasciculus (SLF)
- ■ Inferior fronto-occipital fasciculus (IFOF)
- ■ Inferior longitudinal fasciculus (ILF)
- ■ Arcuate fasciculus (AF)
- ■ Uncinate fasciculus (UF)

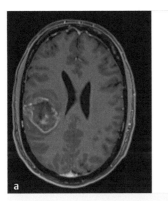
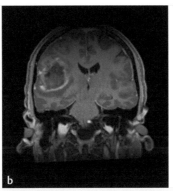
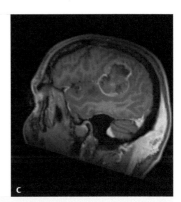

Fig. 11.3 (a–c) The potential functionality and the danger zones.

"Danger-zones." This exercise is very helpful in planning the case. With just a very short analysis of simple MRI scans, you can come up with a reasonable plan:

1. *Analyze the lesion* (based on this standard MRI with contrast series). Answer the following questions (before reading our approach, try to get your own plan).

- Is the lesion eloquent? (Yes, right parietal, near central motor cortex).
- What are the functions at risk?
  a) Functional aspects/vascular conflicts.
     Motor, cortical, and subcortical. Somatosensory system, cortical and subcortical. Optic radiation.

  b) Vascular conflicts: Sulcal arteries providing M1.

Done. You have now collected crucial information for the next step: planning to avoid a deficit.

2. *Run through your IONM options*

The principal options: Awake/asleep/combined. A key decision for planning the monitoring is the decision for an awake or asleep procedure or the combination of both. This is a very complicated and multilayered decision and needs a very individualized approach. A very important factor in this decision-making process is not only the specifics of the individual patient but also the individual settings

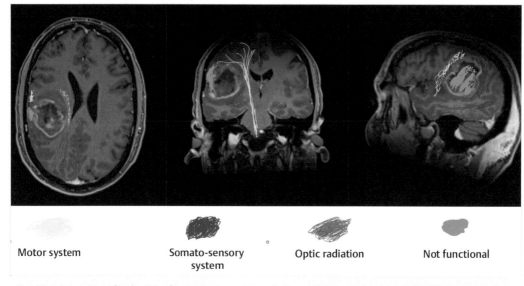

| Motor system | Somato-sensory system | Optic radiation | Not functional |

Fig. 11.4 Approximate localization of motor system, optic radiation, and the somatosensory system according to basic neuroanatomical considerations.

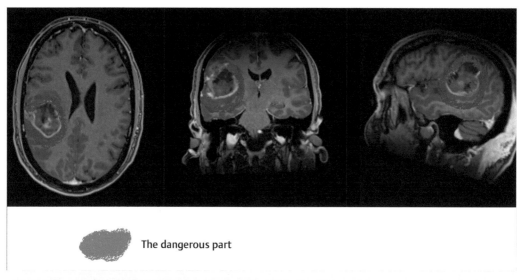

The dangerous part

Fig. 11.5 Area in which an injury to functional tracts is most likely: the danger zone.

in your hospital. If your team does not have yet a large experience in awake surgery, the threshold to perform awake surgery is higher than in centers with a routine approach to awake brain tumor surgery.

Planning the details:
- Which tests can be used to identify these functions?

Principal options are **Motor system** MEPs, transcranial and direct cortical. Motor system stimulation with monopolar stimulator at cortical and subcortical levels. Bipolar stimulation at cortical and subcortical levels in an awake setting.

Somatosensory system (The SSEPs). Test of coordination of movement with bipolar stimulation at cortical and subcortical levels in an awake setting. Induction of dysesthesia by bipolar stimulation at cortical and subcortical levels in an awake setting.

Optic radiation: VEPs. Bipolar stimulation at subcortical level in an awake setting testing for induction of visual field deficits.

- Are these tests in this patient feasible?

According to your files the patient is reported to be "54 years, male, no neurological deficits, otherwise healthy." Probably.

3. Risk assessment

- What are the risks for a permanent deficit due to surgery?

In Germany it is generally assumed that the risk for a permanent deficit in eloquent tumor surgery is around 6%.

- What is the natural course of the disease regarding the occurrence of deficits?

Let's not overcomplicate things: It's for a glioblastoma or a metastasis. Highly aggressive, potentially exponentially growing lesion. The patient will probably lose the functions at risk within months, maybe even earlier.

- Are there alternative treatment options?

Yes, depending on the level of your neurooncological expertise you can identify these yourself. In most semielective cases you will have time to consult a tumor board. Let's assume that both radiotherapist and oncologist are reluctant to treat the not-resected lesion (even if they would have a diagnosis by biopsy).

So, it all depends on you.

Now, however, comes a very important part. You need to evaluate the plan according to the individual situation of the patient and the integration of the patient into the individual social network. At this point medicine turns from scientifically based risk evaluation to art...you will now engage in a very difficult decision-making process, which may often take longer than the surgery itself. We have summarized some thoughts about the decision-making process in ▶ **Video 11.1**.

So, after all your thinking and evaluating:

What is your plan for case 1?

You need to define a plan for the monitoring and define an idea about the possible extent of resection.

We have planned the case as follows:

ASLEEP-AWAKE-(ASLEEP)

Did you consider this case for awake? Right hemisphere? Actually, this is a good case for

awake: Though motor mapping can be done by monopolar stimulation, awake motor mapping gives you the additional functional aspects of complex motor testing.

Though somatosensory cortex can be monitored by SSEPs, line bisection testing is very helpful. Also, the induction of paresthesia could provide you with very valuable information.

Visual fields are probably best tested with 60-Hz stimulation. So, depending on your experience and the patients' attitude consider awake.

Essential monitoring is obviously cortical and subcortical stimulation. You will probably engage transcranial MEP and SSEP monitoring, use a grid electrode, and use ECoG for early detection of spreading or seizures.

- With this setup of the monitoring, what is the resection plan? What is possible?

You have four options:

In sequence of extent of resection:

biopsy < internal decompression < lesionectomy < supramarginal resection.

In addition, for lesions involving the cerebral cortex you have the option of supial resection.

In the presented case it is very likely that you can perform a lesionectomy. If you identify the relevant sulci in the perilesional areas and the cortical areas test negative, you can plan to initiate with a subpial approach. Depending on the subcortical stimulation findings, you might consider a supramarginal resection. Importantly, you need to identify the conditions which allow you to perform the actual ablation. For example, proceeding toward the OR at the infernodorsal part of the lesion is based on the testing of visual fields, hence the cooperation of the patient. If the patient does not cooperate you need to adjust your plan and stop. Or, as you might have discussed with the patient **before**

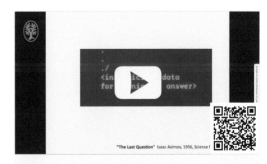

Video 11.1 Decision making process.

surgery, you will go on and sacrifice the visual fields, because the patient prefers a hemianopsia in exchange for a better prognosis.... We strongly advise you to prepare the surgery in a way that will not force you to go through this decision-making process during surgery (**see** ▶ **Video 11.1**). You need a kind of flow chart in your mind and define the plan A-B-C to be adept at the actual neurosurgical neurooncological situation accordingly.

Now, after all this thinking and these considerations it is finally time for putting these all in practice: we are proceeding to the OR.

12 Setting up the Monitoring

In the following video session, we demonstrate the practical details of a typical SSEP (▶ Video 7.2) and MEP setup (▶ Video 7.3). Our group uses the INOMED Isis system; depending on your locally used system, details are certainly a little different. However, principles remain the same.

12.1 Setup of SSEPs

Please review Section 8.3. In ▶ Video 7.2 we demonstrate the setup of SSEPs. In the text below you will find a short outline of the video content.
a) Placement of scalp electrodes is demonstrated. You find the position of Fz, C3′, Cz, Cv1, and C4′ using a ruler as demonstrated.
b) Placement of median and tibial stimulation electrodes.
Remember that the **anode is always distal**, and the **cathode is always proximal**.
c) Getting the baselines.

It is essential to get the baselines before the intervention has started and potential damage is induced. Make it a habit to discuss the findings of the baselines in the team. Important: realize the limitations in the individual setting, (i.e., no tibialis or median SSEPs are detectable). In Section 7.3 (SSEP) we have discussed that the relative position of the electrodes to respective generator is of crucial importance for the amplitude and form of the wave. With the beginning of surgery (▶ Fig. 7.5a and ▶ Video 7.2) the first change you will encounter is very often the displacement of the electrodes relative to the baseline settings. In due course the position of the brain will change and the electrical properties of the system will change (i.e., the impedance due to changes of tissue properties) (i.e., replacement of tumor tissue with fluid or air). In addition, depth of anesthesia will vary, specifically in an asleep-awake setting. Furthermore, temperature changes occur. So, SSEPs are "physiologically" changing and these changes are often not pathological. Real trouble starts with a constant 50% drop in amplitude and a 10% prolongation in latency. Disciplined, direct, and clear communication within the team is necessary to make sure that these changes are immediately communicated.

12.2 Setup of MEPs

Please review Section 7.4 (MEP). In ▶ Video 7.3 we demonstrate the setup of MEPs. In the text below you will find a short outline of the video content.
a) Placement of scalp electrodes: You find the position of Fz, T3, C3, Cz, C4, and T4 using a ruler as demonstrated for the SSEPs.
b) Placement of EMG electrodes: The video shows the placement of the electrodes in the target muscles. In most setups you will limit the number of muscles to less than 10. It is of practical value to order these muscles on the screen in groups: face, arm, hand, leg. This makes it easier for the observer to identify the stimulated area. In most setups you will limit the number of muscles to less than 12. Depending on the localization of the tumor and the subsequent involvement of functional motor areas, you might weight your choice of indicator muscles individually. For tumors in the midline, you would for example prefer the placement of more needles in the leg than in face or upper extremities.
c) Getting the baselines.

As for the SSEPs it is essential to get the transcranial baselines before the intervention has started. As for the SSEPs, make it a habit to communicate the MEP baseline finding within the team. It is crucial that everybody is aware of missing MEP signal of the leg. If you combine transcranial MEPs with an awake procedure, you need to keep in mind that transcranial MEPs need a rather high current and would induce local pain if applied in the awake state. Warning signs: Disappearance, marked amplitude reduction (>50% from baseline), and acute threshold elevation are major criteria that need direct and clear communication within the team.

13 The Surgery

13.1 Case Summary

This is a 34-year-old female accountant. She presented with a focal seizure: postictal anomia and paresis of right hand. As you see her in your office, she has no neurological deficits.

13.2 Planning the Case

Please review the MRI scan (▶ **Video 13.1**) and use the approach described in Section 12.2 to evaluate the surgical procedure. We provide you with some key aspects of the MRI in ▶ Fig. 13.1, ▶ Fig. 13.2,

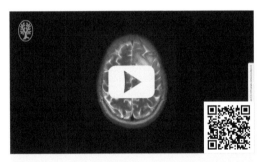

Video 13.1 Film of MRI scans.

▶ Fig. 13.3, ▶ Fig. 13.4, ▶ Fig. 13.5, ▶ Fig. 13.6, ▶ Fig. 13.7. You can use these to analyze the danger points. Please sketch the potential functional areas (both cortical and subcortical) and define your surgical endpoint and strategy, again according to the suggested outline in chapter "Indication for Surgery: Decision-making" before you go watch the video analysis (▶ **Video 13.2**). In this video we guide you through our approach to the case.

In summary we have planned the case as follows:
According to the localization of the tumor we suggest as a minimum:
- ASLEEP-AWAKE-(ASLEEP) (awake essential, rest up to your local preferences).
- 60 Hz stimulation for language and motor mapping.

Optional are:
- Monopolar stimulation as a back-up method in case of noncompliance.
- MEPs and SSEPs as additional adjuncts. ECoG for early detection of spreading or seizures.

13.3 The Surgery

Now we are ready to start the surgery (▶ **Video 13.3**).

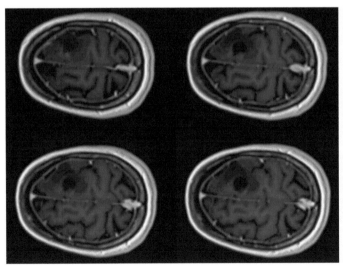

Fig. 13.1 Sequential axial T1 images with contrast enhancement.

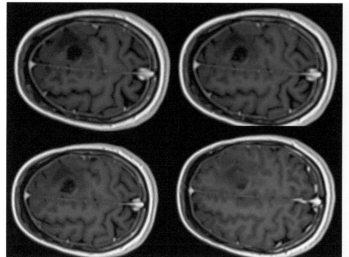

Fig. 13.2 Sequential axial T1 images with contrast enhancement.

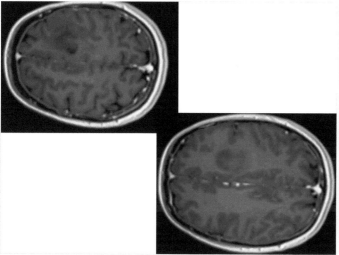

Fig. 13.3 Sequential axial T1 images with contrast enhancement.

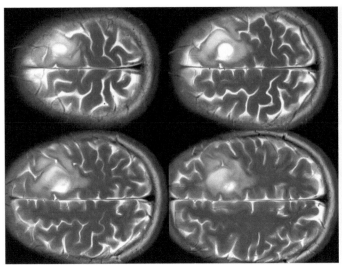

Fig. 13.4 Sequential axial T2 images.

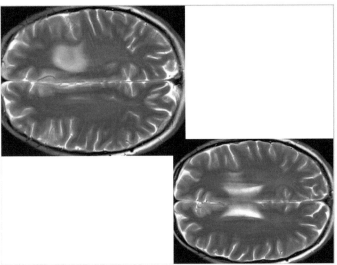

Fig. 13.5 Sequential axial T2 images.

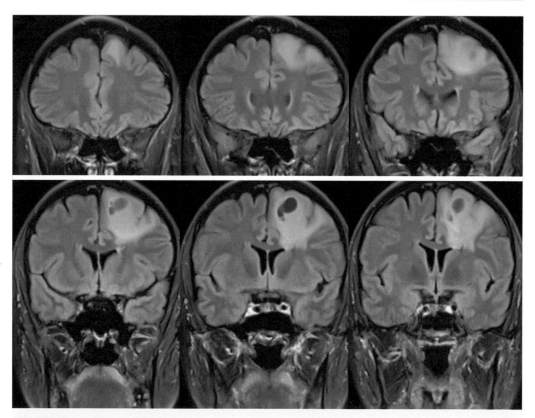

Fig. 13.6 Sequential coronal Flair images.

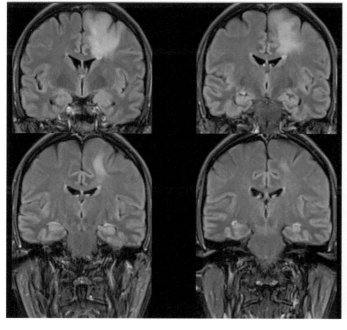

Fig. 13.7 Sequential coronal Flair images.

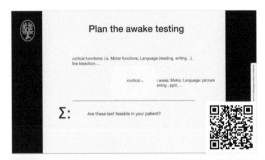

Video 13.2 Analysis MRI.

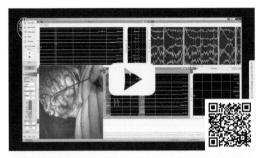

Video 13.3 The surgery.

14 Summary: Key Features from the Video

Here we have summarized the key features of the video for a quick review.

14.1 Getting the Threshold

14.1.1 Monopolar

▶ Video 14.1.

14.1.2 Bipolar

▶ Video 14.2.

14.2 Subcortical Monopolar

▶ Video 14.3.

14.3 Subcortical Bipolar

▶ Video 14.4.

14.4 Subpial Resection

▶ Video 14.5.

14.5 Anomia

▶ Video 14.6.

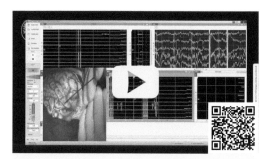

Video 14.1 Monopolar cortical mapping.

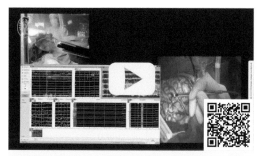

Video 14.2 Bipolar cortical mapping.

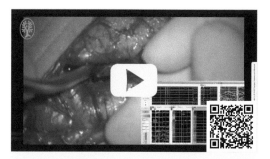

Video 14.3 Subcortical monopolar mapping.

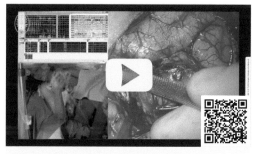

Video 14.4 Subcortical bipolar mapping.

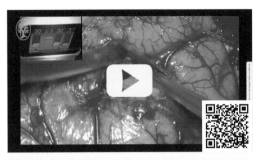

Video 14.5 Subpial resection.

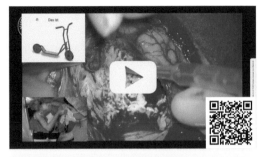

Video 14.6 Stimulation-induced anomia.

15 Epilogue

Neurooncological neurosurgery is always a compromise between preserving functionality and fighting this disabling and deadly disease. We sincerely hope that this book helps to cope with this dilemma. It was not at all intended to give the full picture of neurooncological neurosurgery. In addition to all the efforts in planning, preparing, and performing the surgery, the following adjuvant therapeutic options are of utmost importance. Often these options influence our treatment decision and indications for surgery. It is therefore obvious that a neurooncological neurosurgeon must be familiar with these treatments as well.

In this book we presented the basic principles of how to preserve functions when resecting infiltrating brain tumors. We all sincerely hope that our field will further expand into monitoring options far beyond what was described here. The mere preservation of walk and talk does not satisfy the complexity of the higher cognitive functions at risk. When performing supramarginal resection in patients who will have decades to live with their impairment, we need to expand our evaluation of the outcome to complex testing of neurocognitive performance as well.

A final thought: Despite our best efforts we will not always avoid severe complications. Though we will not suffer from the physical harm that our patient has to confront, we will suffer psychologically. We wish us all to gain the mental strength to cope with these situations and to transform these into the motivation to improve.

List of Abbreviations

- AC: alternating current
- AF: arcuate fascicle
- AG: angular gyrus
- 5-ALA: 5-amino-laevulinic acid
- AP: action potential
- AR: acoustic radiation
- CMAP: compound muscle action potential
- CPS: cortical parcellation system
- DES: direct electrical stimulation
- DC: direct current
- DLS: dorsal longitudinal system
- DLPFC: dorsolateral prefrontal cortex
- IPSP: inhibitory postsynaptic potentials
- E: electromotive force
- ECoG: electrocorticography
- EEG: electroencephalography
- EMG: electromyography
- ERP: event-related potentials
- EPSP: excitatory postsynaptic potentials
- FAT: frontal aslant tract
- Fp: frontal pole
- GBM: glioblastoma multiforme
- HF: high frequency
- HG: Heschl gyrus
- Hz: hertz
- I: ampere
- iMRI: intraoperative MRI
- IFG: inferior frontal gyrus
- IFOF: inferior fronto-occipital fascicle
- ILF: inferior longitudinal fascicle
- IONM: intraoperative neurophysiological monitoring
- ITCp: posterior inferior temporal cortex
- IOG: inferior occipital gyrus
- IPL: inter parietal lobe
- ITG: inferior temporal gyrus
- LOFC: lateral orbitofrontal cortex
- IPSP: inhibitory postsynaptic potential
- LF: low frequency
- MOG: middle occipital gyrus
- MEP: motor-evoked potential
- ms: microsecond
- MTG: middle temporal gyrus
- OR: optic radiation
- P: watt
- POp: pars opercularis
- PPTT: pyramid palm tree test
- PSP: postsynaptic potential
- pMTG: posterior middle temporal gyrus
- pSTG: posterior superior temporal gyrus
- PostCG: postcentral gyrus
- PTri: pars triangularis
- R: Ohm
- SLF: superior longitudinal fascicle
- SMA: supplementary motor areas
- SMG: superior marginal gyrus
- SOG: superior occipital gyrus
- SSEP: somatosensory-evoked potential
- STG: superior temporal gyrus
- Tp: temporal pole
- VPMC: ventral premotor cortex
- VPM ventral posterior medial nucleus
- VOF: vertical occipital fascicle
- VOFA: visual object form area
- V: volt
- VPL: ventral posterior lateral nucleus
- VWFA: visual word form area
- WBRT: whole-brain radiation therapy
- WHO: World Health Organization

Index

Note: Page numbers set **bold** or *italic* indicate headings or figures, respectively.

Index